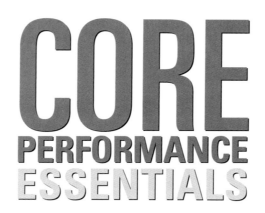

CORE
PERFORMANCE
ESSENTIALS

MARK VERSTEGEN

AND PETE WILLIAMS

CORE
PERFORMANCE
ESSENTIALS

THE REVOLUTIONARY NUTRITION AND EXERCISE PLAN ADAPTED FOR EVERYDAY USE

RODALE

NOTICE

The information in this book is meant to supplement, not replace, proper exercise training. All forms of exercise pose some inherent risks. The editors and publisher advise readers to take full responsibility for their safety and know their limits. Before practicing the exercises in this book, be sure that your equipment is well-maintained, and do not take risks beyond your level of experience, aptitude, training, and fitness. The exercise and dietary programs in this book are not intended as a substitute for any exercise routine or dietary regimen that may have been prescribed by your doctor. As with all exercise and dietary programs, you should get your doctor's approval before beginning. Mention of specific companies, organizations, or authorities in this book does not imply endorsement by the publisher, nor does mention of specific companies, organizations, or authorities imply that they endorse this book. Internet addresses and telephone numbers given in this book were accurate at the time it went to press.

Rodale books may be purchased for business or promotional use or for special sales. For information, please write to: Special Markets Department, Rodale Inc., 733 Third Avenue, New York, NY 10017.

Printed in the United States of America
Rodale Inc. makes every effort to use acid-free ∞, recycled paper ♻.

Photographs by David Zickl
Illustration by Sandy Freeman
Book design by Susan P. Eugster

Library of Congress Cataloging-in-Publication Data

Verstegen, Mark, date.
    Core performance essentials : the revolutionary nutrition and exercise plan adapted for everyday use / Mark Verstegen and Pete Williams.
        p.   cm.
    Includes index.
    ISBN-13 978–1–59486–350–9 hardcover
    ISBN-10 1–59486–350–4 hardcover
    ISBN-13 978–1–59486–627–2 paperback
    ISBN-10 1–59486–627–9 paperback
    1. Exercise.   2. Physical fitness.   3. Nutrition.   I. Williams, Pete, date.   II. Title.
GV481.V47   2006
613.7—dc22   2005024403

Distributed to the trade by Holtzbrinck Publishers

2 4 6 8 10 9 7 5 3   hardcover
2 4 6 8 10 9 7 5 3   paperback

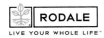

RODALE
LIVE YOUR WHOLE LIFE™

We inspire and enable people to improve their lives and the world around them

For more of our products visit **rodalestore.com** or call 800-848-4735

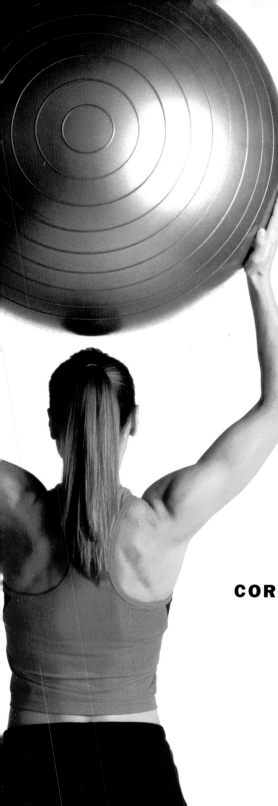

CONTENTS

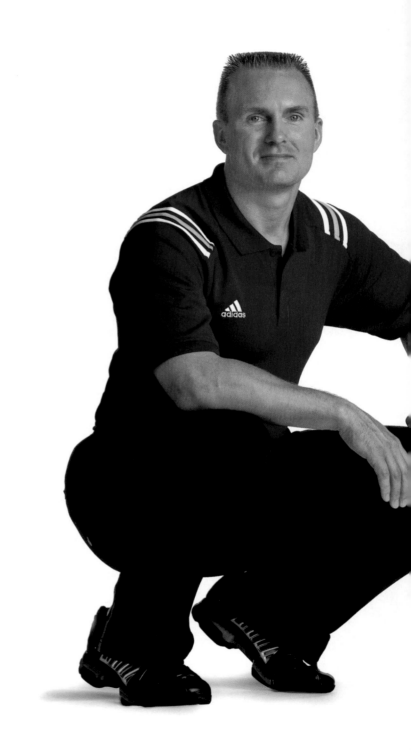

THE GAME OF LIFE

thlete *n.* A person possessing the natural or acquired traits, such as strength, agility, and endurance, that are necessary for physical exercise or sports, especially those performed in competitive contexts.

Everyone is an athlete. Even if you don't play sports, you compete each day in the Game of Life. In order to succeed, you need a strategy to build and maintain the necessary strength and energy to accomplish your goals.

The day-to-day life of a corporate worker, student, or stay-at-home parent is just as physically and mentally grueling as anything you'll find in sports. I work with professional athletes who accomplish tremendous feats, but even the challenges they face sometimes pale in comparison with those that the vast majority of people face every day.

After all, athletes spend most of their time practicing for short periods of competition, and they have the benefit of off-seasons. Most of us have no time to practice; the game is going on all the time. There is no off-season, except the occasional vacation or holiday. The competition never ends.

Not only that, but we risk a lot more than not making the playoffs or taking home the title: Our performance impacts the quality of life and destinies of those we care about most. The stakes could not be higher.

Look at the definition of *athlete* above.

Even if you have never picked up a ball and have no intention of doing so, you need strength, endurance, and agility just to get through daily routines; resist fatigue, frustration, and distraction; and meet the demands of life.

For all the talk of creating washboard abs, counting carbs, and losing weight, many of us have lost sight of what really matters: improving our physical and mental well-being to ensure a productive day-to-day existence, to say nothing of a long and healthy life.

Don't get me wrong; it's important to look great. But why not take the same amount of time and effort that many people invest only in looking good and follow a program that produces not only cosmetic changes but also increases energy, sharpens your mental edge, and reduces and prevents nagging pains in your back, knees, and hips?

Sound good? Here's even better news: You don't have to spend hours in the gym, deprive yourself of tasty food, or acquire an advanced degree in exercise science to understand the regimen.

Core Performance Essentials, as the name suggests, includes everything you need and nothing you don't. The entire program can be done either at the gym or in the comfort of your own home, with only a minimal investment in equipment. Even then, if you don't want to swallow that cost, there are exercise variations that don't require equipment.

You won't be forced to follow a diet program that's aggravatingly complicated, impossible to adhere to, or ineffective. Instead, you'll learn simple principles and recipes that will trim your waistline and food bills while improving your performance.

First, you need to understand that this is a long-term strategy. You'll notice there's no time-stamped subtitle to this book: No "12 Weeks to a Better You"; no "6-Week Plan for Great Abs." This is not a quick fix, a New Year's resolution, or an extreme makeover. I don't want this to be the latest in a series of programs you try, only to give up when you become bored, get too busy, or become frustrated.

After all, even the most successful athletes or businesspeople don't quit after one good or bad season. I'm fortunate to help some of the world's greatest athletes build successful careers, and I want to provide you with similar tools to lead a life of sustained performance and improve your long-term health.

Will it take some effort? Of course it will. You must want to bring out the athlete that's inside of you. But before you start thinking that this process isn't for you, pay heed to the first rule of investing: *Past performance is not indicative of future return.* No matter how bad off you are right now, you're not doomed to poor health and an early exit if you take action now. On the other hand, if you *don't* take action, that past performance—or lack thereof—*will* result in an unhappy future return.

Unfortunately, it's an uphill battle. It's easy to be beaten down by this fast-paced culture; it's easy to think you can eat whatever and whenever you want; it's easy to abandon consistent exercise—or abstain from it altogether—and still feel like you'll come out ahead. So you grind harder, firm in the belief that you can outwork and outhustle anyone through sheer willpower.

Sooner or later, your body will break down due to injury or illness. It's a vicious downward spiral—the harder you work, the more run-down you become and the less energy you have. Nobody can keep up the pace forever unless they have, like the best athletes, a game plan to help them. The idea is to sustain this winning energy level throughout your life.

For instance, let's say you're a successful executive. You wake up in the morning after a short, restless sleep. You hustle out the door and grab a muffin and an expensive, calorie-laden designer coffee on the way to work. While answering e-mail and putting out a few office brush fires, you chug diet soda or more coffee. By lunchtime, you're starving, so you grab some takeout or head to a restaurant for a meal that offers little nutritional value. By midafternoon you're dragging, so you drink more caffeine and get a jolt of sugar from the vending machine. Still, you struggle to get as much work done as you'd like, so you either stay late or take work home, where you eat the first thing you can find, perhaps pizza or pasta. By now, the day is over and your back, as usual, is killing you. You've had no time to exercise. Instead of releasing endorphins and recharging with a workout, you unwind with a few martinis or glasses of wine. You're too exhausted to give quality time to your significant other or kids. It's all you can do to slump in front of the TV for a few hours, grazing on more junk food before collapsing in bed for another short, restless sleep before repeating the process the next day.

Sound familiar?

If not, let's say you're a stay-at-home parent. You're jolted from a brief slumber by a screaming baby, and you stagger around for an hour, dealing with the toddler and getting an older child or two off to school. The youngest commands your attention for most of the day, a whirlwind of diapers, feedings, and playdates. Soon it's midafternoon and it's time to chauffeur the kids to sports, music practices, and other extracurricular activities.

Along the way, you must handle the crush

of household routines, the inevitable home maintenance crisis and, oh yeah, the small matter of feeding yourself. Dinnertime arrives and all you've consumed is coffee and the fast-food lunch on the way back from the playdate. You'd like to work off the extra pounds you've packed on in recent years, but who has the time?

Perhaps you're a student. You wake up too late to have a substantial breakfast, if any, and because you're not allowed to eat in class, you're famished most of the morning. Because of tight budgets, the cafeteria or student union offers little beyond highly processed, high-starch meals, but it does provide soda and vending machines. That burst of sugar carries you through part of the afternoon, but soon, you're struggling to stay awake in class and you're even feeling hungry again.

Even though you're tired, you also feel kind of antsy, like you need to run around. Unfortunately, your school has not offered physical education classes in years. When you finally get home, you're so hungry that you grab the first thing available, which usually is junk food. Homework, phone calls, friends, and e-mail take up the afternoon and much of the evening, which includes pizza or a takeout dinner that your parents brought home.

Remarkably, most people manage to function adequately enough in this fast-forward, time-pressed world to slog through life. But instead of reaching their maximum potential and reaching their goals, they're more like *goaltenders,* deflecting the shots that life fires at them.

The consequences of this defensive lifestyle are devastating. By eating poorly and not exercising, you're not as productive and you accomplish less. You make poor use of your time at work or school, which takes away from the time you can spend with loved ones, to say nothing of your earning potential. Even when you do have time, you're too tired and stressed to offer love and support to the people who matter most.

Still, you manage to achieve a degree of success in work or school and even find some time to spend with your loved ones. But you feel like the mythical Greek, Sisyphus, doomed to endlessly push a rock up a hill, never getting over the top. A little voice in the back of your head, or perhaps a real voice in the form of a doctor or loved one, keeps reminding you to pay attention to your health and get your life in order.

Bottom line: You need to stop playing goalie. After all, even the best goaltenders can't fend off every shot. But this isn't a game: Once your health slips, you're on a downward spiral. And then it's *game over.*

Of course, you're not alone. More than

400,000 people die each year from causes related to poor diet and physical inactivity. That's 17 percent of all deaths. Only tobacco use, according to research by the National Institutes of Health, accounts for more fatalities (435,000 people).

And it's only getting worse. Though the death toll from most preventable causes decreased in the decade between 1990 and 2000, obesity and inactivity deaths went up by a mind-boggling 33 percent. By 2010, poor diet and physical activity likely will overtake smoking as the leading cause of preventable death.

If our health care system is strained now, what will it be like if things don't change? Many companies already have cut back on health benefits, covering only employees and not spouses and children. The ranks of the uninsured grow each year. Many of these people have priced themselves out of individual coverage because of their inactivity and poor eating habits. They're a health crisis away from bankruptcy.

Still, for some people, the realistic prospects of bankruptcy and an early death are not enough to change an unhealthy lifestyle. So let's consider a few more horrors: Inactive people are far more likely to suffer from depression and agonizing back problems; they lose mobility earlier in life and no longer can play sports, lift children, or even walk; and

they're more likely to develop diabetes, which can lead to blindness, kidney failure, and loss of limbs. Worst of all, these ailments are kicking in far earlier than in previous generations.

According to recent research done at Brandeis and Emory universities, per capita health care spending among Americans ages 30 to 50 rose more than 75 percent between 1987 and 2000. We're treating the effects of inactivity and poor diet rather than addressing the causes. According to the Centers for Disease Control and Prevention, the United States spends $1.7 billion annually on medical care, but only 5 percent of this spending is for preventive education and care.

The terrible irony in this crisis is that we soon could see the average life expectancy *decrease,* even though medical technology continues to advance, and even though we know far more about the impact of poor diet and inactivity than ever before.

It's not an exaggeration to say that if this continues, our already precarious health care system will collapse and millions will face bankruptcy and early death. Everyone will feel the impact.

The stakes are high and, unfortunately, the teams are unfairly matched. In one corner, we have overloaded, overworked, overstressed Americans, struggling to balance the demands of work and family. They find it difficult to exercise, plan, and prepare healthy meals, and take a proactive approach to life.

In the other corner stands a powerful opponent: 21st century America. Its roster includes wealthy fast-food marketers bombarding us with pitches for their unhealthy, seductively convenient foods, many made with unnatural, high-fat substances.

The opponent's roster has other strong players, including vast cable television universes, the Internet, and video games looking to grab our attention. There are cash-strapped school boards forced to cut physical education classes and raise money by allowing vending machines and fast-food sponsorship of school lunches.

It's time to level the playing field—and I'm here to help. For the last 15 years, I've had great success working with athletes at all levels, from those who have won Super Bowl, World Series, and World Cup championships to the thousands of folks who read my first book, *Core Performance.*

If you missed that book, that's okay. In fact, look at *Core Performance Essentials* as both a prequel and a sequel to *Core Performance.* If you're one of those people facing the challenges discussed above, this is the perfect starting point. This book is designed for time-pressed adults for whom *Core Performance* might be a little too taxing. It's for kids who

want to get off the couch and establish some good habits at a young age. It's for the person who has never engaged in much physical activity, but who is looking for an effective, easy-to-understand place to start. It's even for the person who wants to augment an existing program or freshen up a routine that's grown stale.

It's also a sequel for *Core Performance* readers who, for whatever reason, no longer have as much time to commit to a more extensive regimen. This is an abbreviated program that provides the most benefit in the least amount of time.

But this is much more than just another diet and nutrition program. Too many books give you those components, figuring you'll find a way to make it work. Together, we're going to create a new lifestyle around your existing structure and provide you with the motivation and tools to make your better habits permanent.

After all, you have commitments etched in stone in the form of family and work. So you have to establish this athletic mindset and be ready to go, because this isn't just a tennis match or round of golf. The consequences of falling short in life are so much greater than they are in sports.

In short, this book is for you, the competitive athlete in the Game of Life. Here you'll find everything you need—the Core

Essentials—to create a positive lifestyle based on core values, physical activity, and healthy eating that will fuel you toward success in every aspect of your life. Your goal is *to live longer and live better.* It's to weave this system into a healthy lifestyle that will be at the heart of everything you do.

Consider *Core Performance Essentials* your new playbook. It's your life—are you ready to get in the game?

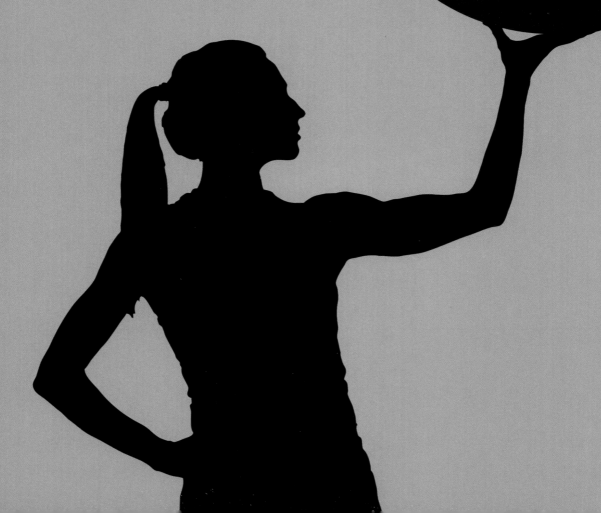

MINDSET

NUTRITION

MOVEMENT

RECOVERY

THE
CORE
MINDSET

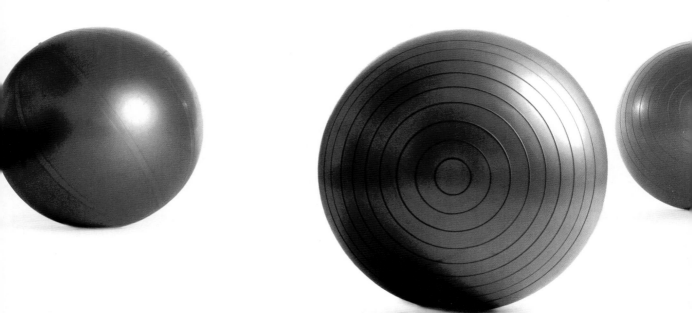

WHAT'S AT YOUR CORE?

So, now you're thinking we're going to launch into a nutrition and workout discussion, right? Not so fast. Before we do that, we need to tweak your lifestyle and thought process. If you start a diet and exercise program without a big-picture lifestyle master plan, you're doomed to fail.

The idea behind this program is that everything starts from the core. We want to build our lives from the inside out, not just at the superficial level, like so many other programs.

Core is a popular buzzword. Most people think it refers only to your abdominals, and countless books and articles have been written on how to produce six-pack abs.

But your core, from a strictly physical standpoint, is much more than just your abs. As we'll discuss later in the book, the core refers to the midsection of the body—from hips to shoulders—and is the basis for all movement.

If you look at this as just another diet and exercise program, you will have a difficult time producing long-term change. That's why I want you to think broader. Think of this as an integrated lifestyle system with four components, the four parts of what I call the Core Essentials: Mindset, Nutrition, Movement, and Recovery.

When embarking on a new program of nutrition and exercise, you will be far more moti-

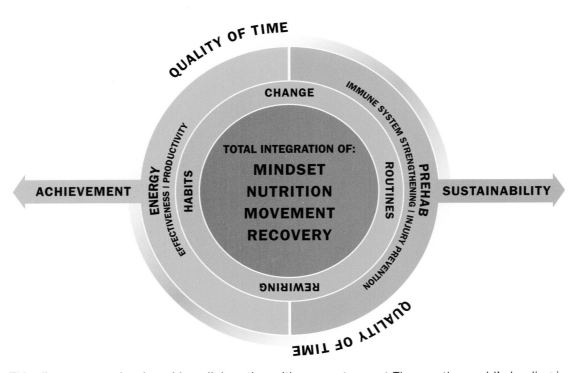

QUALITY OF TIME

CHANGE

IMMUNE SYSTEM STRENGTHENING | INJURY PREVENTION

EFFECTIVENESS | PRODUCTIVITY

ENERGY

HABITS

ACHIEVEMENT

TOTAL INTEGRATION OF:
MINDSET
NUTRITION
MOVEMENT
RECOVERY

ROUTINES

PREHAB

SUSTAINABILITY

REWIRING

QUALITY OF TIME

This diagram was developed in collaboration with our partners at Tignum, the world's leading institute for executive excellence.

vated if you take a step back and define what drives you. So, don't look at our Core Essentials sphere above as an abstract concept. Instead, think of it as a Super Ball. When I was little, I'd take one of those tiny red Super Balls and slam it as hard as I could on the driveway. It seemed like it would go 50 feet in the air, bounce, and then go another 20 feet. I marveled at the power of this simple 10-cent object smaller than a golf ball. Indeed, the reason a golf ball or baseball can travel such a great distance is because there's the equivalent of a Super Ball at its core.

We want to create a Super Ball in your own core, not just through nutrition and exercise but by rewiring your mindset and incorporating recovery into your lifestyle. Let's take a brief look at each of these four components.

MINDSET

The simple fact that you picked up this book suggests that you have, to some degree, the proper mindset to make the necessary changes in your life.

I once had the wonderful opportunity to chat

4

with John Wooden, perhaps the greatest college basketball coach of all time. He told me that he always looked for players who were not just willing, but *eager,* to do what it takes. Until a player was eager to become the best he could be, Wooden said, there was no use in him showing up for practice.

On the surface, that might seem like a minor distinction. But think of the relationship that most people have with their jobs. They're willing to show up for work—after all, they presumably need the money—but not really eager to do so. As a result, their performance isn't exemplary—it's just good enough for them to keep their jobs.

(Of course, there are other contributing factors. People who suffer from depression, anxiety, arthritis, diabetes, high blood pressure, and other ailments lose much of the productivity they once had.)

This epidemic of "presenteeism" is sweeping our nation, and not just in the workforce. Technically, people might be present on the job—or with their families or when taking part in activities they once actively enjoyed—but they're not engaged, not thriving, not striving. They're bogged down with the demands of life, suffering from ailments, sleepwalking through their days with no light at the end of the tunnel. The thought of doing the same thing for the next 15 or 20 years, with no increase in quality of life, can be immobilizing: No wonder so many people suffer from depression. If you don't have a game plan to handle the demands of life, to create energy, you'll never lead the life you want to lead.

In the next chapter, we'll help you *rewire* your mindset so you can create *change* and develop *routines,* formulating great *habits* that will last a lifetime. Most diet and exercise programs assume that if you eat right and get into better shape, everything else will take care of itself. Well, aside from a lucky (and dedicated) few, that only works for the short term, and most of us need a game plan to keep us going. After all, even the most physically gifted athletes cannot succeed unless they have mentally addressed everything they will face in competition. Developing the proper mindset will help prepare you for everything that comes your way.

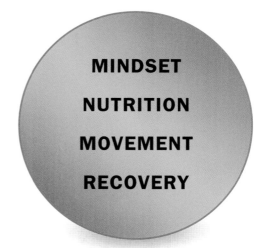

MINDSET

NUTRITION

MOVEMENT

RECOVERY

NUTRITION

If you want to create that core Super Ball, you have to fuel your body properly. Even if you do nothing else (i.e., exercise), eating right will go a long way toward protecting your health.

I've never understood why diet books outsell fitness books by such a large margin. Apparently, more people would rather deprive themselves of food through dieting than take a proactive approach to their health through a combination of nutrition and exercise.

You won't find that here. What you *will* find is that together, we're going to change your approach to eating. Instead of living to eat, we're going to *eat to live*. It's that simple. Instead of using food to change your emotional state or deal with stress, you're going to use it to fuel your body for maximum performance. It's not just about losing weight or looking good in a bathing suit—both of which you'll accomplish, by the way.

Instead, you're going to use food to fuel your success and sustain your energy level. Not only that, but by planning to eat properly and putting a game plan in place, you'll also save time and money.

MOVEMENT

I hesitate to use the term *exercise* because it's come to mean something with a definitive beginning and end: *I'm going to the gym now, so therefore it's time to exercise.*

I prefer the term *movement* since it's more indicative of an active lifestyle, even outside the gym. I'll show you ways to work your body in any situation, whether it's sitting at your desk or sitting in an airplane. It can be as simple as taking the stairs instead of the elevator. Try to take every opportunity to move your body, not just during formal exercise. Think of your entire life as a potential workout.

Proper movement is what will give your "Super Ball" its power; otherwise, you're more like a softball. There might be a solid core in there somewhere, but it's covered with so many layers of string that it has minimal impact. With this program of proper exercise, you'll develop those "super" powers.

RECOVERY

"I give 110 percent every day."

If I really meant that, I'd be lying. The reason I'd be lying is that nobody can give 110 percent—or 100 percent, for that matter—every day. The body, mind, and soul won't allow it.

There are people who work 18-hour days, 6 days a week, and never take a vacation. What's the point? I know there are people who love their work—I'm fortunate to be one of them—but if I didn't have the time to enjoy the fruits of my labor then I'd be wasting my life.

Not just that, but it's impossible to maintain such a furious pace without your body breaking down. Throughout this program, you'll learn the importance of recovery, or what I like to call *regeneration.*

A starting pitcher in baseball, for instance, cannot throw full-throttle every day. He needs to rest 3 or 4 days between outings. Yes, he can throw lightly between outings, and some relief pitchers can pitch short stints most every day. But it's impossible for any pitcher to go all-out for lengthy periods of time every day without risking injury. Regeneration is necessary.

Regeneration applies to everything: Exercise, nutrition, and mindset. You can't work out hard 6 days a week; your body will break down. So, we've constructed this program with hard days and easier "regeneration days" that allow you time to recover.

The same is true with nutrition. If I instructed you to eat nothing but healthy foods, 7 days a week, you'd never be able to follow the program. So I'm giving you one day a week to eat however you please. It allows you to take a mental break and reward yourself. (By the way, there's also a 3-week indoctrination period to help you build up to eating healthy for most of the week.)

Regeneration also applies to your mindset. The primary purpose of a vacation is for your mind to recover from the grind of everyday life. We need to build these breaks into our lives in order to come back even stronger.

Think of how that Super Ball continues to bounce high six, seven, or eight times. We want to bounce back from the demands and pitfalls of life, returning stronger each time. Recovery is the ability to come back up to that level as rapidly as possible, no matter how poorly the ball bounces. Recovery allows us to create constant momentum.

These four components—Mindset, Nutrition, Movement, and Recovery—do not operate independently. This is an integrated program that will permeate every aspect of your life. So let's begin with establishing that proper mindset.

Chapter 1 Summary: *Core Performance Essentials* is not just a diet and exercise program but an integrated lifestyle system that incorporates four elements of the Core Essentials sphere. Those components are Mindset, Nutrition, Movement, and Recovery. By working all four aspects of the system, you can produce the energy and structure to thrive in the Game of Life.

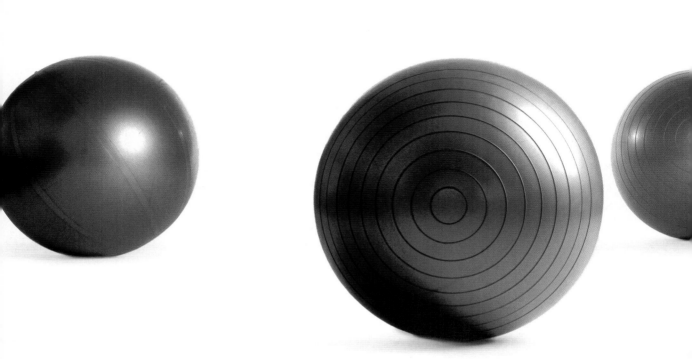

CHAPTER 2

THE CORE SELF

Most people get through days with a false sense of accomplishment. They do a great job of playing goalie, handling tasks, and juggling duties at a furious pace. At the end of the day, however, are they really better off? Have they invested in the long-term health of their bodies through physical activity and proper nutrition? Have they gone on the offensive, guided by core values, and worked toward personal goals that will bring about lasting change? Or have they merely endured another day of making a living?

Think of yourself for a moment as a powerful force for producing change in the lives of family and friends. What have you done each day to build your powers? Not just in your career, but in terms of making yourself into the person you want to be? What are the core values and goals that drive you?

Unlike in sports, the difference between winning and losing in this game is not always clear. How can it be if we haven't defined the rules we play by? Do we really know what will make us "successful"? Do we let society dictate to us its view of success? Is it really about accumulating financial wealth, looking like a

THE MEANING OF SUCCESS

What is your definition of success?

What roles do you play at home, at work?

What drives you?

What would the other people you touch through your various roles say about you today, as opposed to what you'd like them to say about you in a eulogy?

What do you need to do in order to create the change so that they will say what you would like to hear in your eulogy?

magazine model, or having the most friends on the block? Is it just about getting that next promotion, getting the kids to their next appointment on time, losing those 10 pounds we swore we would? Or have we not truly examined what will mean everything to us when we look back on our lives?

We need to make a deeper examination. You have unique roles in life, and I'd venture to say that there is nobody out there who plays just one part. When an athlete comes to me, I need to know which sport and which position he plays before we even think about defining his goals and the success he hopes to attain. Without knowing what role he plays on his team, we can't accomplish anything together. Similarly, there are a lot of positions you could play. Through "The Meaning of Success" and "What Roles Do You Play in the Game of Life?" exercises, described here, you are going to define your positions and responsibilities in the game.

Once you've done this, we need to do the same thing that I do with superstar athletes: evaluate you, based on where you are and what you need to perform your position well. And then, together, we'll create sustainable change that allows you to do a better job playing your positions and supporting your team.

This process should change your mindset, giving you tangible goals based on who you are and whom you support, not on how much you make or how you look. Throughout this book, we'll give you the game plan that will help you live up to the high standards you should—and will—set for yourself. It will be the best investment of time you'll ever make. Take a moment now and create your own meaning of success through the exercise above. You can write in the book, but perhaps it would be more effective to use a separate sheet of paper that you can access more easily.

This is a deeply personal exercise, but my

advice for everyone is the same: Dream big. For me, success is directly correlated with the depths of my relationships with the people I care about most. I will have been successful if I have helped improve the quality of their lives. If I've done that, then my life will have stood for something special and will continue to live on in those people long after I'm gone.

My definition of success also would be to fully use what God and my parents gave me, to the best of my abilities, and to carry on those family values. Perhaps the biggest value I learned growing up was the notion of service, to make sure that I lead by example in all areas of my life and to help others in a way in which they can do the same. Through hard work, passion, honesty, and the courage to lead the life that I've dreamed of, I can be-

come successful. I will not accept anything less from myself.

Even if you've never defined success, I'm guessing deep down that you know what your vision of real accomplishment is and what you want to create. We all have core values that we do not want to compromise. Every day, we're faced with choices to make the right decisions, and it takes strength and courage to do that as you make your way toward your best self.

But you need to have that direction. For our purposes, it doesn't matter what your definition of success is—what's important is that it will point the way to fulfillment. This is your inspiration to get in the game.

Through the exercise below, ask yourself what you need to fulfill each of the roles you

WHAT ROLES DO YOU PLAY IN THE GAME OF LIFE?

What are your roles?

What do you need to do for each of these roles? What will be the definition of success to improve quality in each one of these roles in life?

Ask yourself: What will make you feel successful in the areas of mental, physical, and spiritual development?

What will make you feel successful in the important role you play for your spouse or significant other?

What do you need to do to be successful in your role with your family—as a son or daughter, brother or sister, father or mother?

What role do you fill with your friends? How can you fill this role more successfully?

What is your role with your colleagues at work, at school, in the organizations of which you're a part?

play. What role do you play for your spouse or significant other? What roles do you play to make the relationship special? What does your position require? When discussing what they need to play their roles effectively on the field, athletes mention things like speed, strength, and agility. When you're talking about making a relationship work, it's about listening and being understanding. It's about creating and spending meaningful time together.

Once you've defined the roles you play, ask yourself what other people would say about you in these roles. Would your spouse say that you don't make enough time, or that you are not intimate enough when you do? What would you want your spouse or significant other to say?

What would your family say about you? Would parents or siblings say that you don't take the time to call? Would your children say that you don't have time to read a bedtime story? Perhaps they would say you're conscientious about making calls outside of birthdays and that you readily engage in random acts of kindness. You're the person they can turn to for advice, help, or support.

What would your friends say about you? Would they say that you're there for them when they need you? Or would they say that they're tired of hearing about all your problems, about how life has been unfair? How about your coworkers? Would they say you're a nice person?

Would they think you're productive and effective at work or someone who drags down the office?

If you work in an office or go to school, would your colleagues say that you goof off too much? Or have you found the happy medium, able to buckle down when you have to, but not taking yourself too seriously? Are you known for laughing and having fun or for being stressed out and holding on too tight?

In short, what do you want people to think or say about you? Go back to each of the roles listed above. Are you setting a good example? Are you comfortable with the way you're perceived?

So, what does any of this have to do with nutrition and exercise? In a word: everything. You need to identify these core values before you can embark on a physical transformation. It will give you added motivation to work toward your long-term success plan, but, more important, you'll come to recognize that this isn't just about you—you're undertaking this transformation to better serve and elevate the people you care about most.

The concept of being **guided by core values** in a program of energy production, exercise, and proper nutrition in the interest of achieving long-term success and elevating the lives of others is what I call the **centered self** or *core self*. Keep in mind that your core is the center of your own world, but that doesn't mean things revolve around you. Instead, use that strong core to elevate others.

Sounds simple enough, right? Unfortunately, we've become such a self-centered culture that we fail to look inside ourselves, into our cores, for deeper meaning and guidance. Whatever happened to all that discussion after 9/11 about how we'd take a broader view of ourselves, strip away the superficial nonsense, and focus on what's really important?

That didn't last long. Now we have the national plague of reality television and extreme makeover shows promising immediate solutions for everything from our faces to our homes. We walk around with cell phones glued to our ears, oblivious to everyone else. We're obsessed with six-pack abs, celebrity, and overnight stardom. There are books and magazines devoted to "trading up" in everything from clothes to cars to homes. We've created superstars out of people like Donald Trump and Paris Hilton, mostly for being rich and self-centered.

This might seem like a digression, but it speaks to the core (pun intended) of what we're trying to accomplish in this program. If you look at your diet and exercise program as just another quick-fix, must-have accessory or luxury item, this is not going to work.

Among the many reasons why most nutrition and exercise programs do not produce lasting change is that people view their health as something to be renovated, a remodeling project with a definitive beginning and end. They want the fastest, easiest possible solution, and, failing that, there's always plastic surgery and liposuction.

People tend to make changes from the outside in. But unless you make fundamental changes, overhauling your mindset, it's just short-term, until one day you wake up not quite sure who you are, where you've been, or where you want to go.

Life isn't about finding yourself; it's about *creating* yourself. Who do you want to be? That's the great thing about sports. Kids pretend they're someone else who plays a certain way. They grow up emulating the qualities and abilities that they like. That's how they shape their development—by mimicking the people who do it best.

We're all works in progress, and that process of *real* self-improvement should never stop. The biggest question any of us needs to answer is: *Who do you want to be, and why?* What's important to you? Is it family, friends, and relationships? Is it exercise and staying active? If you had all the money in the world, what are the things you would do? What fulfills you?

Once we've defined success and considered the roles we play, it's easier to start looking at ourselves from the perspective of the **centered self as opposed to being self-**

centered. By embarking on this process, you're going to be better able to lift your friends and family, but it starts with you.

Understand that you're building from the inside out, mentally and physically. If you take care of that and work this process to improve the quality of your life through nutrition and exercise, then you'll be on your way toward fulfillment—and that's what leads to lasting change.

It's the difference between being a show car and a race car. You might see one of Dale Earnhardt Jr.'s cars at a trade show or auto dealership. It looks like "Little E's" car and has all the right decals, but there's nothing under the hood. The real race car, with the high-performance engine and modern technology, is someplace else.

Like that race car, we want to build our core to perform for specific purposes, to sustain higher levels of energy and well-being. That's the type of person we're trying to build—not that empty shell of a show car.

The centered self is guided by deeper meaning, and it looks to elevate others. The self-centered person thinks, "I just want to look better." If that's the case, why not just get chest implants and liposuction? It's a lot less time-consuming than training.

As we've made clear, looking good isn't motivation enough to establish a long-term, life-changing game plan. You'll lose weight and look better, perhaps temporarily, but once that's accomplished, it will be tougher to motivate yourself to continue. But if you're working for a higher purpose, it's easier to focus on that as constant motivation.

You have to feel a deeper, emotional connection to your health; otherwise, it's just another project to complete and cross off the list. But if you can feel the changes that improved health produces, it will serve as constant motivation, whether it's the immediate endorphin rush after a workout, the sustained energy you feel all day long from eating correctly, or the greater financial security you create for your loved ones.

But, of course, it's not enough to say, "Okay, starting today, I'm going to be less self-centered and focus more on my core values and helping those who matter most to me." That's not a bad mission statement, but you need to execute the strategy, driven by the exercises on pages 10 to 11. Otherwise, you'll just get caught up in the whirlwind of daily routines and end up playing goalie again. You either produce energy or you take it away, and if you take it away, you risk ending up as one of those 400,000 people who die every year from obesity and inactivity.

Think of those examples from earlier in the book of the business executive on the corporate treadmill; the harried, stay-at-home parent; and the frazzled student. Or just look at yourself in the mirror. Take an inventory of how you're prematurely aging. Besides the extra pounds, you're dehydrated, which ages the

CORE SUCCESS STORY
"The Gift of Health"

NAME: MIKE DIXEY

AGE: 36

HOMETOWN: SAVAGE, MINNESOTA

Mike Dixey's life was literally spiraling out of control. In 1999, he got out of bed after celebrating his birthday the night before, and he fell to the ground. The room was spinning. "I wouldn't have been worried if I had been drinking," Dixey says. "But I don't drink."

Over the next 5 months, Dixey underwent MRIs and CT scans and visited neurologists. He was diagnosed with vertigo, though doctors didn't know what was causing it.

"The only thing they knew was that my eyes were not seeing what my brain was registering," Dixey says. "Anytime I'd make a quick change of position, I'd have trouble. I'd wake up and think the ceiling fan was running, even though it wasn't on."

And that was when he *could* sleep. Dixey spent nights tossing and turning, unable to fall into a restful sleep. Traveling on airplanes was difficult. He maintained a strict regimen of medication. Doctors told him he would have to live with the condition for the rest of his life.

Because he was also dealing with the chaos of being a new father, getting up constantly at night to help with baby feedings and eating whenever and whatever he could, he packed on 30 pounds. Many nights, he ate pizza or Chinese takeout at 10:30 or later.

Dixey knew that he was a heart attack waiting to happen, what with a long history of heart disease in his family. His father has survived a heart attack and his mother, triple-bypass surgery. Three aunts underwent quadruple bypasses. Dixey's paternal grandfather died young from a heart attack.

Throughout his twenties, he had worked out using bodybuilding-style routines. That did little to change his overall fitness, and he underwent knee surgery and suffered from back and shoulder pain. "I never realized that I had reached a plateau long ago," he says. "I wasn't seeing any benefit."

It's not that Dixey didn't understand the challenge; he works as a physical therapist and has a vast library of fitness literature. In 2004, he began the Core program, eating properly and performing movement-based exercises.

"It's the first program I had found that combined flexibility, strength, and rotator cuff movements. Everything about it made so much more sense."

Dixey lost 21 pounds in the first 12 weeks of the program and dropped 32 pounds overall. Soon his back, shoulders, and knees were pain-free. He was able to touch his toes for the first time since childhood, and he made plans to play in a 35-and-older baseball league.

Most important, the vertigo all but disappeared. He still feels a mild form occasionally if he is stuck in traffic with cars whizzing by from the other side. But he's off medication and sleeping peacefully—or at least as well as any parent with two kids under the age of 6 can expect.

"I look great, and more important, I feel great," Dixey says. "I'm looking forward to playing baseball and being back in control of my life. That's the greatest gift this program has given me—the gift of great health."

skin more. You have poor posture from sitting so much and not exercising, so you look slouched over, older, and less confident. Since you don't get enough sleep, you have bags under your eyes, get sick more often, have less energy, and look perpetually run-down. You find it increasingly difficult to concentrate and be productive at work. Perhaps you're on medication, or you self-medicate with alcohol or drugs, which only exacerbates your problems. No doubt your sex drive isn't what it once was.

I know you mean well. Against all of these odds, you've been successful at work and at home, to one degree or another. In a sense, you've sacrificed your body for the good of the team, your loved ones. You're doing everything possible to be that centered self. But if you don't make immediate changes to re-verse this downward spiral, your team is going to suffer some big-time losses.

Think of someone you know who has died young from a heart attack or an illness brought about by an unhealthy lifestyle. Maybe this person had it all—wealth, family, an enviable career. But none of it means anything because they couldn't stay around to affect the lives of others.

You can't buy health, which is vital to becoming a centered self. By placing a premium on relationships, core values, and long-term goals that elevate others, you come to the conclusion that health is the vehicle that drives the system.

It's impossible to accomplish anything without health. If you're constantly tired, run-down, and playing goalie, unable to take care of yourself, how can you ever think about oth-

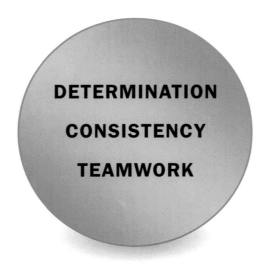

DETERMINATION

CONSISTENCY

TEAMWORK

ers? It even breeds resentment to the point that you might think, "I'm killing myself here and nobody appreciates it!"

We need to learn to be better teammates. Here's where we can learn from professional athletes: They can inspire us with their dedication to the team and, every so often, to a much higher cause.

Let's consider three concepts from sports that apply:

Sport, at its essence, is people overcoming obstacles. Athletes have the **determination** to stare down adversity with unwavering confidence in themselves, whether it's the 1980 U.S. Olympic Hockey Team dispatching the Soviets in Lake Placid or the 2004 Boston Red Sox coming back against impossible odds against their greatest rival, the New York Yankees.

Athletes reap the rewards in the form of great fame and fortune. You toil more anonymously, trying each day to reach your goals and realize your aspirations. Regardless, like a world-class athlete, you have to stay steadfastly focused on your goals, and you have to remain confident that you can attain them. At the end of the day, you have to ask yourself if you've moved closer—even by just a few inches—to achieving a specific goal.

The key is to be consistent. **Consistency** can be a misleading term since it's often associated with repetition, complacency, and mediocrity. But for our purposes, look at it as the consistent pursuit of greatness. After all, there are plenty of recreational golfers who can play one round on a PGA course and shoot a 68. But can they do it consistently? That's the difference between world-class performance and having a good day. Great golfers have become so consistent that even on their worst days, they're still pretty darned good. When you can sustain that high level and build upon it over the course of a career, that's when you achieve greatness.

We want to take that same approach, especially in the workouts we'll discuss later in the book. We don't aspire to consistent mediocrity, so that we end up complacent and doing the same routines over and over, never getting better. We want to seek consistent greatness.

Teamwork is perhaps the greatest motivating factor in establishing that consistency. Even in individual sports such as tennis and golf, athletes have a small army of supporters. There are coaches and trainers, family and friends, and all manner of support staff.

Being part of a team carries an enormous responsibility. You never want to be viewed as the weakest link or as letting your teammates down. Instead, you want to raise the level of play of the entire team to another level, regardless of your position.

Even if you don't play sports, you're a member of at least one team: your immediate family. Perhaps you've reached the point where you've spun off and formed an expansion team, a family of your own.

Those are important teams, and you must play your position extremely well in order to support those around you. That means you have to be a little selfish in finding time to take care of your body. This is where a lot of people go wrong: They rationalize eating poorly, working longer hours, and failing to exercise. "I don't have time to exercise or eat right. I must forge ahead and work harder. My family is counting on me!"

It sounds almost heroic. But though your intentions are good, you're letting down the team. It's like the guy who tries to play on a bum ankle or knee, getting by at 50 percent. It's impressive, and sometimes adequate, but sooner or later he's going to break down, and he'll bring the team down with him.

The same holds true in life. If you have struggled with nutrition and exercise, it's time to start thinking of the impact on your most important team. Professional athletes get replaced all the time. There's always someone out there who's younger, faster, cheaper, and so players get released, they get traded, and eventually hang up their spikes and sneakers. But you're irreplaceable.

So, in order to make sure you can be there for your team, let's start by properly fueling your body, the vehicle for your success. We'll start in the next section with the Core Nutrition program—everything you need to know to maintain a high-performance diet. Though the nutrition section comes before the workout, I don't mean to imply that one is more important than the other, though I understand why people place more importance on eating right than working out. After all, everyone has to eat to survive, so why not just diet? People figure they don't *have* to exercise, though it's tough to live a healthy lifestyle on just diet alone. You get so much more benefit out of a nutritional program by exercising—and vice versa. Remember that what and how you eat is only *part of* building your centered self.

In fact, you'll find that when you combine a proper nutritional program with a core-based workout that emphasizes functional movement, you'll be in a position to accomplish most anything.

I've made the workout program in this book as easy and time-sensitive as possible, but if you find that there are times when you can't follow it, then at least stick to the nutrition portion. That alone will improve your health significantly. But let's make this a perfect progression: You established your core values and centered self in this section. Now, let's change our eating habits and put together a workout program to maximize our success.

Throughout this book, you'll hear from people who managed to do just that.

Chapter 2 Summary: Successful people are driven by core values that permeate every fiber of their being. By defining success through these values and applying it to each of the roles you play in life, it's possible to accomplish anything. Unlike many people in our self-centered society, we each want to be a centered self, or core-centered, using these values as fuel for our daily lives and to obtain long-term goals.

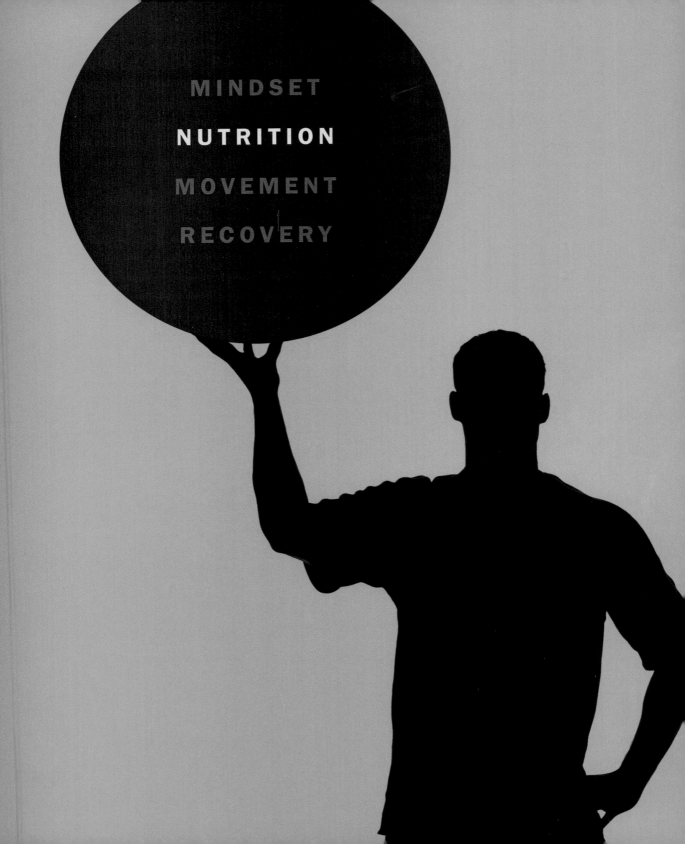

CORE
NUTRITION

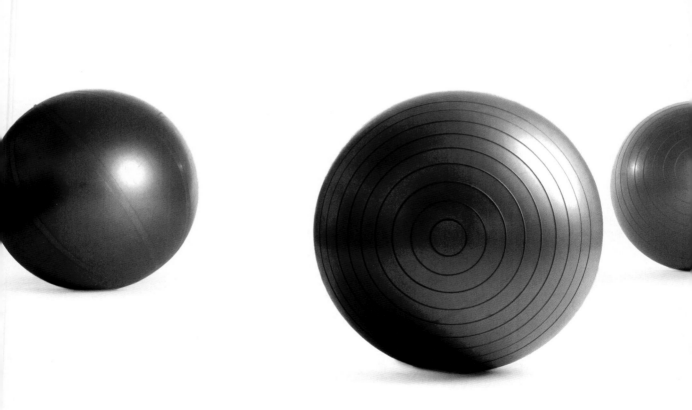

TWO-MINUTE WARNING

You might think nutrition doesn't matter. Maybe you've gotten along just fine with a little extra weight. Unfortunately, the older you get, the more those surplus pounds take their toll. You're more vulnerable to heart disease and diabetes, you have less energy, and you don't accomplish as much as you otherwise could. No matter how successful you are, I'm sure you'll agree that you could do even more if you were in better shape.

The bottom line is that, left unchecked, your body is a crisis waiting to happen. Consider this your two-minute warning. Fortunately, there's still time. Joe Montana and John Elway fashioned Hall of Fame football careers out of their last-minute comebacks. In that spirit, we're going to show you how to turn your nutrition plan around quickly.

Maybe you already have a good plan in place. At this point, you have a game plan to build your centered self. You've installed an athlete's mentality and know to build everything from the core. But think of yourself as the general manager of a new franchise with far greater resources.

Now we're going to literally transform our

CORE NUTRITION ASSESSMENT

Have you stocked your pantry, refrigerator, and freezer with foods that you can quickly put together for a nutritious meal or snack any night of the week?

Have you stocked your office cabinet or vehicle with similar foods?

Do you ever react to your body by grabbing caffeine or snacks at the vending machine to "keep you going" throughout the day? (And have you ever considered walking around the office or doing pushups instead?)

When you're hungry and searching for your next meal, do you often decide to pull through the drive-thru because of time constraints?

bodies through nutrition. You will learn how to eat and drink to fuel your body for optimal energy and production. In short, the Core Nutrition game plan is a great way to maximize energy, lose fat, gain lean mass, and save money and time.

But before you get started with the program, please complete the Core Nutrition Assessment above.

The purpose behind these questions is to illustrate that at the core of great nutrition are *environment* and *planning,* things as simple as the power of your pantry, refrigerator, freezer, and a well-stocked desk at work. So, if you answered no to either of the first two questions and yes to either of the last two questions, you're setting yourself up for long-term health problems.

As with the rest of this program, I want you to think like an athlete about nutrition. After all, you're certainly competing in a high-stakes game, and you need a powerful, turbo-charged body that burns fuel efficiently and produces the consistent energy you'll need to reach your full potential.

If you consume soda, hot dogs, and fast food regularly, you'll end up among the ranks of the obese, putting yourself at an extreme disadvantage in everything you do. Oh, you don't agree? Well, in 2003, filmmaker Morgan Spurlock tried to eat nothing but McDonald's for an entire month. A healthy, fit young man when he started, he packed on more than 20 pounds in a couple of weeks. Soon he was walking around in a daze, with little energy and an addiction to the food. His doctors and nutritionists told him that if he did not stop the McDonald's diet, his vital organs might shut down.

Spurlock's movie, *Super Size Me,* inspired McDonald's to eliminate its largest portions from its menu. He deserves praise for educating the public on the dangers of fast food and how it's so shamelessly marketed.

We're up against the wall when it comes to eating properly. Everywhere we turn, someone's trying to sell us quick, convenient, cheap junk food. They will stop at nothing, labeling food "low fat" or "low carb," even as they load it up with high-fructose corn syrup and trans fats, two fat-producing substances we'll discuss in-depth later.

From now on, be an educated consumer when it comes to playing the food game. Be a smart player. Whether it's ordering a restaurant meal or reading a label for contents, you need to make the best decision for your healthy lifestyle, which you'll learn how to do in the next chapters.

Most important, you have to plan and prepare. Otherwise, you're at the mercy of what's out there, most of which is not good. The number one reason people don't eat properly and sabotage their fitness programs is because of shoddy planning.

When it comes to nutrition, like everything else in this program, you have to think for the long term. It's easy to rationalize eating unhealthy food—after all, you're hungry and you need to eat something. You're not *that* overweight. Perhaps you didn't want to be rude to your hosts, refusing that high-fat dish they served. Besides, it really tastes good!

Each time you face such a dilemma, stop and ask why you're on the brink of eating whatever junky food is at hand. Are you letting emotions drive your decisions? What could you do to make a better decision? Even if you are stuck in a fast-food restaurant, what's the best choice available?

After all, those few moments of junk-food-induced pleasure end quickly. So, too, does the value of the food in terms of producing energy. Soon you'll be hungry again. There's also the negative long-term impact that the unhealthy food will have on your body.

Make a positive investment instead. Each time you eat properly, remind yourself that you're not only giving yourself the energy needed for optimal performance, but you're also investing in your long-term health—to say nothing of helping yourself feel and look better.

I know the prospect of embarking on a new nutrition plan is scary. Maybe you've tried other diets. You've counted calories or carbs, followed the Atkins or Zone diets—whichever one happens to be trendy this week. Perhaps you've experimented with miracle supplements that supposedly help you lose weight or gain energy. None of them have proved to be a complete, long-term solution. Instead, they set you up for failure.

The challenge with most programs is that they tend to address the symptoms—too much weight and a lack of energy—rather than the problem, which is poor nutrition in general.

Under this plan, you're going to have five or six small meals or snacks a day, which means you get to eat something every 2½ to 3 hours. If you eat often, your body becomes a more efficient energy-producing machine. (Ask yourself what burns more wood, a hot fire or smoldering coals?) Not only that, frequent eating keeps you from overeating. If you know you're going to have something in a few hours, you'll be less likely to overeat—and less likely to be extremely hungry.

The reason most people don't eat properly is because they don't plan ahead. Remember the athletic mentality? If an athlete does not prepare, looking ahead to what he will face in the game, he's doomed to fail. The same is true with eating. If you don't plan, you end up devouring whatever you can grab.

The process of stressing out over where and when to eat is unhealthy, a problem made worse by the junk you inevitably consume in such a state. As a result, you end up increasing body fat and decreasing lean mass, which defeats the purpose of following the Core Movement program in the next section. Not only that, but eating on the run is also expensive. It costs more, not just in terms of the money you lay out at the restau-rant, but in terms of the damage it does to your health.

As we formulate our game plan, let's take a look at the strengths of our opponent, which really aren't strengths at all but widely held misconceptions.

Eating right is time-consuming: On the contrary, eating right saves time. If you have your meals plotted out for the entire day—or the entire week—you'll save hours each week.

Compare the person in your office who brings lunch from home with the person who has to go out to a sit-down restaurant or unhealthy fast-food franchise. The one who brought lunch from home already has saved a minimum of 15 to 30 minutes, and most likely he'll eat a healthier alternative.

I'm not advocating eating at your desk, though in many hectic offices this is reality. If that's the case, you'll fall behind by ducking out to locate lunch. Not only that, but if you have lunch handy, you're less likely to go hungry and rush out to find the first option available, which usually is a losing battle. One easy way to get a jump start on the week is to do all of your shopping on Saturdays or Sundays, which will help you plan out your meals for the week. This is a great way to be really proactive about your choices.

Eating right is expensive: Actually, eating

"I proved the pharmaceutical rep wrong."

NAME: PAT BINKLEY

AGE: 36

HOMETOWN: SEATTLE

Like a lot of new parents, Pat Binkley struggled to find the time to exercise. With a hectic schedule as an executive for a software company and three children under the age of 6, he saw no openings in his schedule.

Still, he knew he had to find a way. His cholesterol was 270. He carried 170 pounds on his 5-foot-9 frame, which, although hardly obese, "was bad weight," according to Binkley. "I had a double chin and a pretty good spare tire going. I even had man boobs."

Binkley joined a gym, began leaving home at 5:30 for morning workouts, and followed the Core program religiously. He made it home to shower and have breakfast before the kids got out of bed.

"There was no way I was going to find an hour in the day anywhere else," Binkley says. "I'm sort of a morning person anyway. I had to do it. Now it's become my sacred time."

Binkley overhauled his diet. He began looking at the supermarket in terms of zones, focusing on the outer aisles, where produce, meats, and healthier foods are housed. He learned how to study labels for nutrition content. Most important, he made sure he grazed on the right kinds of food throughout the day.

"I'm more aware now that I can't let my body go into starvation mode," he says. "I try to eat something during those long in-between periods. That gives me more consistent energy all day long and allows me to eat less during what used to be three larger meals. If you don't have those in-between-meal snacks, you're going to make poor decisions and overeat later."

Since starting the program in March 2004, Binkley has felt stronger. The spare tire has begun to disappear. His wife has noticed the difference. Then there are the intangible rewards: "The thing that surprised me the most is how much more energy I have for the kids," he says. "I can pick them up and even hold two or three of them at a time. Before, my back would be hurting. Now I can put the heaviest kid up on my shoulders. I can wrestle with them, ride bikes, play catch—be there for all of those quality-time things that I couldn't really enjoy before."

These days, Binkley's weight is down to a lean 157. His cholesterol is below 200. He recently ran into a pharmaceutical salesperson who had told him it was impossible to reduce cholesterol by 10 percent—let alone 35—by diet and exercise alone.

"I thought I'd need [to take] drugs," Binkley says. "I still wonder if I'm going to be able to make this a lifelong routine as opposed to something I did for a couple of years in my midthirties. But when you feel good and can be there for your kids, that's all the motivation you need."

right *saves* money. If you've planned your day and week, chances are you'll eat out infrequently, which saves a lot of cash. When you have not prepared ahead of time—like the reactive office worker above—you're more likely to grab the first option available, regardless of cost.

Let's not forget the greater cost of eating out: the cost to your health. Researchers at the University of Massachusetts found that eating more than one-third of your meals in restaurants increases your risk of obesity by 69 percent.

Eating right means I'll only be consuming bland, tasteless food: This is a big misconception. It's easy to prepare meals that not only are good for you but taste good as well. There are dozens of delicious foods, condiments, and spices that we'll discuss in the coming pages that will help you to eat meals that are both healthy and delicious.

Fast-food restaurants thrive because they perpetuate all these myths. After all, they provide tasty, inexpensive food, quickly. That food might be cheap, though it's still not as inexpensive as planning and preparing meals. Moreover, low-nutrient, high-sugar, high-fat foods rob us of energy, produce nasty mood swings that affect our relationships and decision-making, and increase body fat. In the long term, this may decrease your quality of life and overall well-being.

We have come to believe that, even though we work hard, we have no control over our lives and are not making the most of our potential. It's a brutal downward spiral. We make the excuses that there's not enough time, that we're in too much pain, that we don't have enough energy, or that spending time with family is more important than taking time to plan and stick to a healthy game plan.

It all starts with the food we eat. No matter how diligently we follow the Core Workout—or any program—it won't matter unless we properly fuel our bodies.

Did you know that most people eat poorly 80 percent of the time and healthfully the remaining 20 percent? Most of the time, they consume high-calorie foods low in nutrients and fiber.

We want to flip that equation, striving to eat healthfully at least 80 percent of the time. It's unrealistic to think that we'll be perfect, no matter how hard we plan. Plus, we're building in a "free" day to eat whatever you want, within reason. That's one-seventh of a week right there.

So, let's sound the two-minute warning. No longer will we be nutritional goalies, scooping up everything that comes our way. Instead, we're going to deflect these shots, letting in only those foods that will fuel us well, provide energy, and contribute to long-term health.

Chapter 3 Summary: The key to eating properly is planning. By stocking the pantry, refrigerator, and freezer with healthy options at home, you avoid eating poorly at home. By keeping an office cabinet supplied with similar foods, you avoid having to grab caffeine or snacks at the vending machine to keep you going. Eating healthful meals and snacks saves money and time.

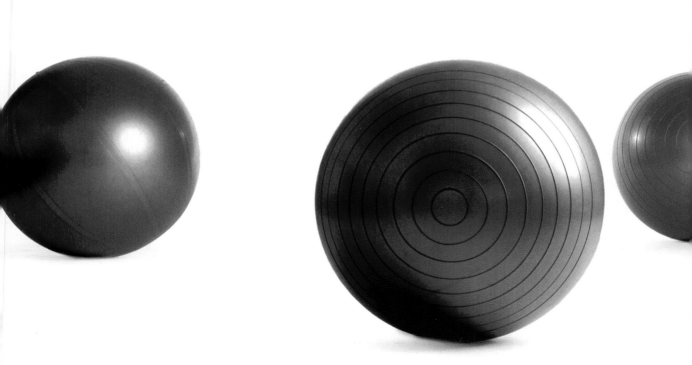

CHAPTER 4

REVIEWING THE RULE BOOK

We've become accustomed to eating a certain way because, well, that's the way it's always been. We accept certain nutrition rules as inalienable truths when many of them are misconceptions. In this chapter, we're going to review and rewrite the rule book, inserting new strategies to properly fuel our bodies.

CORE NUTRITION STRATEGY #1: EAT OFTEN

We've been taught to get three square meals a day, avoid between-meal snacks, and not eat after dinner. No wonder we tend to feel bloated from overeating, hungry and lethargic between meals, and starved before bedtime.

To control appetite, regulate your blood sugar level (which improves concentration and helps regulate appetite), and build lean body mass, you must eat five or six small- to medium-size meals or snacks each day. That means you need to eat, on average, every 3 hours. Think of yourself as "grazing" throughout the day, instead of sitting down for three massive meals.

Frequent eating is like constantly throwing wood on the fire. Digesting food cranks up your metabolism and burns more calories every time you eat. When you eat only occasionally, the fire smolders and dies. A hot fire, on the other hand, burns wood continuously.

You can eat six times a day regardless of your job or lifestyle. The six "meals" are not going to be long, sit-down affairs. Three of your meals could be a piece of fruit and a handful of nuts. Take what you might have previously considered a large lunch and save part of it for midafternoon.

On the days you work out, which might be every weekday, you'll consume pre- and/or post-workout recovery shakes. And since you're eating more often, your traditional breakfasts, lunches, and dinners should be lighter.

If we don't eat often, the most readily available substance for the body to consume is muscle. Many people believe that the first thing the body eats away is fat. But that's a misconception—in point of fact, the body is remarkably resistant to fat loss and will turn to its lean muscle mass first, keeping that stored fat in reserve as long as necessary.

Many people try to get thin by not eating. They deprive their bodies of nutrients and, while they might look healthy, they may have dangerous blood profiles and a high ratio of fat to lean muscle. Their bodies are what I call "skinny fat" (others call them "skinny soft"). They look skinny, but they actually have a high percentage of body fat.

The last thing we want to do is lose lean mass. After all, we're going to be working hard to build this lean mass, which produces power,

stabilizes joints, promotes movement, and is critical for optimal performance. We lose a pound of lean mass per year after our mid-twenties, so it's imperative to take action to maintain this lean mass and function.

To that end, we must eat often, which brings us to our next strategy . . .

CORE NUTRITION STRATEGY #2: CONTROL THE GAME CLOCK

Everyone has a different schedule. But like a good football, basketball, or hockey team, we're going to use the clock to our advantage.

Here are three ways to schedule your six meals, depending on whether you work out in the morning, during lunch, or after work. I've also included some menu suggestions and a schedule for those who compete in early evening ball games.

Option A: For Those Who Work Out Before Work/School

6:15 a.m.

Pre-workout shooter (See "'Shot Clock' Pre- and Post-Exercise Nutrition" on pages 36 to 37.)

6:30 a.m.–7:30 a.m.

Workout

7:30 a.m.

Meal #1 (**Breakfast:** Egg-white omelet with vegetables)

10:30 a.m.

Meal #2 (Shake or snack)

1:30 p.m.

Meal #3 (**Lunch:** Tuna with fat-free mayonnaise and/or celery, lettuce, and tomato on rye bread, or as a salad)

4:00 p.m.–4:30 p.m.

Meal #4 (Shake or snack)

7:00 p.m.–7:30 p.m.

Meal #5 (**Dinner:** Grilled salmon with vegetables and whole wheat couscous)

10:00 p.m.–10:30 p.m.

Meal #6 (Shake or snack)

Option B: For Those Who Work Out during Lunch Hour

7:00 a.m.

Meal #1 (**Breakfast:** Oatmeal and a *small* piece of deli meat)

10:00 a.m.

Meal #2 (Shake or snack)

11:45 a.m.

Pre-workout shooter

Noon–1:00 p.m.

Workout

1:00 p.m.

Meal #3 (**Lunch:** Chicken breast on sourdough, pumpernickel, or rye bread with vegetables)

4:00 p.m.

Meal #4 (Shake or snack)

7:00 p.m.

Meal #5 (**Dinner:** A grilled cut of lean red meat with brown or wild rice and vegetables)

10:00 p.m.

Meal #6 (Shake or snack)

Option C: For Those Who Work Out after Work

7:00 a.m.

Meal #1 (**Breakfast:** A bowl of Kashi cereal with blueberries)

10:00 a.m.

Meal #2 (Shake or snack)

1:00 p.m.

Meal #3 (**Lunch:** Chicken breast on a bed of spinach or lettuce with sliced tomatoes, a small sprinkling of nuts, and olive oil for dressing)

4:00 p.m.

Meal #4 (Shake or snack)

5:30 p.m.–6:30 p.m.

Workout

6:30 p.m.

Meal #5 (**Dinner:** Lean pork in Shake 'n Bake seasoning with vegetables)

9:30 p.m.

Meal #6 (Shake or snack)

Option D: For Those Who Work Out or Compete in the Early Evening

7:00 a.m.

Meal #1 (**Breakfast:** Low-fat, low-sugar yogurt with flaxseed oil and/or oatmeal)

10:00 a.m.

Meal #2 (Shake or snack)

1:00 p.m.

Meal #3 (**Lunch:** Lean turkey on rye, pumpernickel, or sourdough bread with vegetables or a salad)

4:00 p.m.

Meal #4 (Shake or snack)

6:00 p.m.

Meal #5 (**Light dinner:** Seasoned grilled swordfish fillet with vegetables)

7:00 p.m.

Workout/Game/Competition

9:00 p.m.–9:30 p.m.

Meal #6 (Post-workout shake or snack)

This might seem as if you're eating a lot, but you're not, if you consume smaller portions. We've become accustomed, especially in the United States, to eating super-size servings. Fast-food restaurants now refer to them as "value" sizes, to make you feel good about getting more for your money, even though you're still pigging out on junk.

One of the best ways to avoid overeating and maintain a healthy metabolism is to pay attention to portion sizes. By eating smaller portions more often, you give your body a better chance to digest and get all of the nutrients from the food. A piece of fish or meat should be about the size of a deck of cards, and a serving of starches (rice or pasta, for example) should be the size of a baseball. On the other hand, it's tough to eat too many vegetables.

Here's one simple way to eat the proper portions: Use a smaller plate. Who says you have to use a 12-inch plate like you're loading up at an all-you-can-eat buffet? We've grown accustomed to thinking that we're not eating a full meal unless we fill up a whole oversize plate. By using a smaller one, it's easier to eat the proper portion.

Most people eat dinner around 7:00 p.m. and don't eat again until breakfast. That's as much as 12 hours without food, so your body gets through this extended fast by tapping into your lean muscle for nourishment. But, if you have that last snack at 10:00 p.m. and breakfast at 6:00 a.m., you can minimize the effects of the fast while getting a full night's sleep.

That final snack or shake at 10:00 p.m. should include something high in protein, since that helps build lean muscle. You also want fiber and essential fats (such as found in fish or flaxseed oil). For many people, a protein shake or high-protein meal-replacement bar might be an easy option. Fruit with lean protein and healthy fat is a good choice as well, since it's full of antioxidants and jump-starts the regenerative process. So an ideal bedtime snack could be a protein shake with a teaspoon of flaxseed oil and a handful of blueberries. Or perhaps a glass of fat-free milk and a handful of almonds.

The bottom line is that by eating every 2½

to 3 hours, you'll maintain consistent energy levels and turn your body into an efficient, fat-burning machine.

CORE NUTRITION STRATEGY #3: BUILDING "REAL DEAL" MEALS

When planning meals, it's vital to consider the role of carbohydrates, proteins, fats, and fiber. Contrary to popular belief, they all must be included in an effective nutrition plan.

Carbs are our fuel, though the amount consumed must be proportional to your level of activity. If I fill up my car's gas tank, drive 5 miles and then fill it up again, it's going to overflow. But, unlike with a car, you might not realize you're overfilling your tank and contributing to a higher level of body fat.

Generally speaking, the more active you are, the more carbs you want to consume. Since most people tend to be more active in the morning and afternoon, it makes sense to eat the majority of your carbs earlier in the day.

Every meal should include fruits and vegetables because of their fiber and nutrient densities. I recommend that you "eat a rainbow often," which refers not only to the bright colors of fruits and vegetables but also to the fact that you should eat six small meals and snacks a day. Typically, your plate should consist mostly of colorful, high-fiber vegetables. There should be a piece of meat or fish the size of a deck of cards, and, if you like, a fist-size portion of

brown rice or whole wheat pasta. There also should be some "good" fats in the form of, say, salmon or olive oil. (We'll discuss fats in more detail later in this chapter.)

When in doubt, remember to "come back to Earth"—given a choice between something processed and something organic, go with the non-processed option.

Scouting Report: Carbs

Strengths: Provide energy for muscle function and act as the primary fuel for the brain. Some carbs, such as whole grains, fruits, and vegetables, are rich in fiber, helping to control appetite, slow digestion, and improve the health of your heart. Fruits and vegetables contain powerful antioxidants, helping to protect the body from the cell-damaging effects of free radicals.

Weaknesses: Processed carbs, such as white breads, pastas, and baked goods, provide little nutritional value and are converted quickly to sugar and easily stored as fat.

Ideal Players:

● Fruits and Vegetables: Apples, asparagus, avocados, beets, bell peppers, black beans, blackberries, blueberries, broccoli, brussels sprouts, cantaloupe, carrots, celery, cherries, cucumber, eggplant, field greens, grapefruit, green apples, green beans, green peas, honeydew, kiwifruit, mangoes, mushrooms, oranges, papaya, peaches, pineapple, plums, pomegranates, raspberries, red grapes, romaine lettuce, snap peas, soy-

"SHOT CLOCK" PRE- AND POST-EXERCISE NUTRITION

You never want your body to be deprived of key nutrients, especially when you work out. Yet many people exercise first thing in the morning on an empty stomach. Don't get me wrong; exercising is a great way to start the day. In fact, that's my only time to work out. But eat something before your workout, even if it's just half an apple or a pre-workout "shooter," which is something like a watered-down glass of orange juice with a scoop of whey protein or simply a glass of water with the scoop of whey.

Whey gets into your system quickly, which is especially important for eating prior to or immediately following a workout. I also recommend a post-workout recovery shake, such as Myoplex or Myoplex Lite, produced by EAS. These prepackaged, convenient shakes contain an effective ratio of proteins, carbohydrates, and fat, and are loaded with fiber, vitamins, and minerals. Since the shakes can be made by mixing water with a scoop or packet of powder in a covered plastic container or blender, they make a quick, easy, and portable snack that won't spoil.

Ideally, you should have a shake right after the workout. At that point, your cells are wide open and screaming for nutrients, and by drinking one of these shakes, you expedite the recovery process and maximize the lean-muscle growth.

Recent research has also shown that the pre-workout shooter may produce an effect equal to a traditional post-workout recovery shake. The pre-workout shooter works its way into the bloodstream to give the muscle exactly what it needs at the earliest possible moment.

Because everyone who reads this will be on a slightly different schedule, there's no one-size-fits-all routine I can offer. But if you remember the priorities—eating often and incorporating a pre-workout shooter and/or a post-workout recovery shake or meal—you can plan your day accordingly. (I'll even customize this to your exact schedule at our Web site, www.coreperformance.com, to remove any guesswork.)

SCOUTING REPORT: (WHEY) PROTEIN SHAKES

Strengths: A by-product of cheese manufacturing, whey (pronounced "way") includes many essential amino acids that boost the immune system and promote overall good health.

---

beans, spinach, squash, strawberries, sweet potatoes, tomatoes, watermelon, yams

● Breads, Cereals, and Grains: Brown rice, Cheerios, couscous, Kashi, oatmeal, pumpernickel bread, quinoa, rye bread, sourdough bread, whole wheat bread

Bottom Line: Non-processed, fiber-rich, colorful carbs are essential to a healthy lifestyle. Eliminating carbs produces sluggishness, along with long-term negative health effects. Carbohydrates are your fuel and should be consumed in proportion to your level of activity. Remember: A portion of carbs should be about the size of a baseball.

Weaknesses: None.

Ideal Players: Whey protein is found in post-workout recovery mixes, so you will be getting them in your shooters, but you also might want to try adding an extra serving to your diet. The flavored powder tastes great sprinkled on oatmeal or mixed with milk, water, or juice.

Bottom Line: Whey provides numerous health benefits for a small investment of time and money.

Whey is quickly digested, which makes it great for eating around workouts. Many protein shakes combine whey protein with another type of slower-releasing protein, casein. This mixture provides a combination of fast- and slow-releasing proteins, which allows for complete coverage over the 2½- to 3-hour window between meals.

Protein shakes accelerate workout recovery. You can buy shakes in a ready-to-drink (RTD) container, or easily make them yourself by mixing water with a scoop or packet of powder, so they're a quick and easy snack that's rich in lean protein but devoid of bad fats.

I strongly recommend Myoplex, a whey shake made by EAS, as well as many of their other ready-to-drink products. In the interest of full disclosure, let me say that EAS is one of my company's strategic partners. Could you get the same value in similar products from other manufacturers? Perhaps, though I've been in this business for more than 15 years and I've yet to find more effective products. Not only that, but EAS was also the first company to meet the stringent "accuracy in labeling" standards of the NSF (National Sanitation Foundation) and the "banned-substance free" certification standards of the NFL and the NFL Players Association. I'm also a big fan of Amino Vital products. Yes, they're another one of my company's strategic partners, but I daresay that no other sports drink products on the market so effectively deliver the amino acids your body needs for greater fitness and higher performance.

PRE-WORKOUT SHOOTER IDEAS

Either of these "recipes" will provide a great pre-workout boost.

- ½ cup orange juice + 1 cup water + 1 scoop whey protein
- 1 scoop EAS Endurathon + 6 to 12 ounces water

Bottom Line: Always have a post-workout shake or meal with carbohydrates and protein to aid recovery. Add a pre-workout shooter to speed up your recovery even more.

Low-Carb Diets

If you go on one of those diets without carbs, it's like taking a sponge and wringing the water out. You'll lose the water weight, but as soon as you eat carbs again—and you will at some point, because you need energy to function, and you can only go so long without carbs—then that sponge is going to fill up with water. Research shows that the weight will come right back, and with a vengeance; people often gain back all the weight they lost while following a diet that severely reduces carb intake—and more. As with all dieting, you'll likely lose some of your lean mass in the process.

Overall, carbs are an important part of your diet when you consume them relative to your activity level and within the context of the glycemic index and glycemic load, which we'll address below.

Scouting Report: High-Fructose Corn Syrup (HFCS, a form of carbohydrate)
Strengths: None. It tastes good, which only helps food manufacturers. When low-fat and fat-free diets became a national obsession in

EVALUATING CARBOHYDRATE "SPEED" WITH THE GLYCEMIC INDEX STOPWATCH

Popular diets have brainwashed millions into believing that carbs are bad, period. If something is high in carbs, don't eat it. Virtually every restaurant chain and food manufacturer has transformed its menus and products to eliminate carbs.

Actually, carbs are essential for healthy living. Good carbs provide energy and are rich in fiber, and many are packed with powerful protective antioxidants.

So how can we tell the good carbs from the bad? Let's start with the *glycemic index,* which is a measure of how a single food will raise your blood glucose level. For instance, let's compare broccoli with cotton candy. If you eat 100 empty calories of cotton candy, it dissolves quickly in your mouth and is absorbed immediately, sending your blood sugar level sky-high. Give kids a high-glycemic food such as cotton

candy, and they'll bounce off the walls. Even adults feel a sugar rush.

The problem is that you crash quickly and end up feeling sluggish. Your body then craves more sugar. Cotton candy, not surprisingly, has a very high glycemic-index number.

If you eat 100 calories of nutrient-dense broccoli, however, your body will have to work much harder to break it down. Eating raw or slightly cooked broccoli (which retains its crunch) causes you to really *chew* it, while your mouth releases powerful digestive enzymes to help initiate the breakdown before the broccoli hits your stomach. It's going to take your body more time to digest. The benefit is that the sugar from the food will be released into your bloodstream more slowly, giving you steady energy over a longer period. In addition, fiber-rich

broccoli sates your hunger and will, ahem, keep things moving through your system. Broccoli, therefore, has a low glycemic-index number.

As a result, you should eat foods with low or moderate ratings on the glycemic index. But since we rarely eat just one food at a time, we need to think about the body's overall glycemic response to everything on our plates. If you eat a high-glycemic food at the same time as some low-glycemic foods, the overall *glycemic response* is moderate, which is fine.

Another way to think of this is in terms of the *glycemic load,* which is computed by taking the food's glycemic index and multiplying by 0.01, then multiplying that total by the number of calories per serving. I don't expect you to actually do this, but the thing to remember is that the larger the

the 1980s, manufacturers removed fat from their products. Instead, they dumped additional high-fructose corn syrup into it to make up for the appealing taste that the fat had provided.

Weaknesses: The reduced fat and added

sugar in foods high in HFCS send blood sugar sky-high before crashing quickly. This process makes us hungry for more food, and so we will likely exceed our total caloric needs.

As a result, HFCS creates a vicious cycle,

portion of high-glycemic carbs, the higher the glycemic load will be.

Generally speaking, the lower the number on the glycemic index, the more natural the food will be. Your body has to work to get the nutrients out of these foods, and that's good, because that gradual release helps regulate blood sugar. Look for natural foods with more color and fiber, since they control appetite, have more nutrients, and improve your cardiovascular system.

By controlling your blood sugar, you're regulating the hormone insulin. If you're constantly jacking up your blood sugar by eating only high-glycemic foods, crashing back down, and then eating more high-glycemic foods, you create a vicious cycle that results in increased calorie consumption and body fat levels, obesity, and perhaps even diabetes.

The reason we see so many overweight children these days, aside from an utter lack of exercise, is that much of what we feed them are high-sugar, high-glycemic processed foods that wreak havoc on blood sugar and provide little nutritional value. Not only does this have serious health implications, it can also lead to attention deficit disorders and wild mood swings that affect development and performance.

GLYCEMIC INDEX OF POPULAR FOODS

LOW	MODERATE	HIGH
Sweet potatoes	Mashed potatoes	Baked potatoes
Yams	Sweet corn	Doughnuts
Green peas	Bananas	Waffles
Black beans	Cantaloupe	Bagels
Oatmeal (not instant)	Pineapple	Raisin bran
Peaches	Hamburger buns	Graham crackers
Oranges	Muffins	Pretzels
Apples	Cheese pizza	Corn chips
Grapefruit	Oatmeal cookies	Watermelon

forcing consumers to eat more high-glycemic food to maintain that blood sugar rush, rather than eating foods the body needs to control appetite and blood sugar level.

According to a study published in the *American Journal of Clinical Nutrition,* Americans ate an average of about half a pound of high-fructose corn syrup in 1970. By 1997, we were consuming up to 62½ pounds each, annually!

Ideal Players: None. Unfortunately, this sweetener is in everything, from soft drinks to ketchup to canned soup. It's also prevalent in juices, breads, and every manner of processed food. Is it any wonder that obesity rates have soared over the last 3 decades?

Bottom Line: There's nothing wrong with a little high-fructose corn syrup. If it's listed first or second in the ingredients list, glance at the product's nutrition facts label to see how much sugar is in the product, and if it's more than 8 grams per serving, find a different brand or, if necessary, a healthier substitute. Generally speaking, avoid products with HFCS.

Scouting Report: Fiber
(A form of carbohydrate)
Strengths: Improves gastrointestinal health and function and helps prevent colon cancer, regulates blood sugar, and promotes long-term cardiovascular health by reducing cholesterol.

Weaknesses: None.

Ideal Players: Fiber is found in beans, many fruits, leafy green vegetables, legumes, oatmeal, whole grain products, as well as in supplement form. Sprinkle oat bran fiber on meals or in your shakes to improve their nutritional value.

Bottom Line: Fiber, found mostly in carbohydrates, is essential to overall health. People who follow low-carb diet plans deprive themselves of this vital source of nutrition.

Scouting Report: Proteins
Strengths: Builds, maintains, and restores muscle. Responsible for healthy blood cells, key enzymes, and strenghtening the immune system.

Weaknesses: In order to build muscle, protein must be consumed with enough carbohydrate calories to provide the body with energy. Otherwise, your body will tap into the protein for energy. Certain forms of animal proteins contain high amounts of saturated fats—for instance, heavily marbled beef.

Ideal Players:

● Fish: Anchovies, calamari, cod, flounder, grouper, halibut, mackerel, mahi mahi, salmon, sardines, swordfish, tuna canned in water, tuna steak, sushi

● Shellfish: Clams/mussels, crab, lobster, oysters, shrimp/prawns

● Poultry: Chicken breast (if skinless), extra-lean ground turkey, turkey breast

● Meat: Buffalo, filet mignon, flank steak, 93% lean ground beef, 96% fat-free ham,

London broil, lean pork loin, tri-tip, top and bottom round of beef, venison

● Legumes: Black beans, lentils, pinto beans, refried beans (if fat-free), soybeans (edamame)

● Dairy products: Cheeses with less than 2% fat, low-fat cottage cheese, Egg Beaters and other egg substitutes, egg whites, fat-free milk, and low-fat, low-sugar yogurt

Bottom Line: Adequate protein intake, spread throughout the day, is vital to long-term health.

I recommend that you consume 0.6 to 0.8 grams of protein per pound of body weight. If you weigh, say, 180 pounds, you would want to shoot for between 108 and 144 grams of protein per day. Generally speaking, the leaner and more active you are, the higher your protein intake should be on that scale.

That might sound like a ton of protein—and it is a significant amount—but consider how much protein is in common foods such as the ones listed below.

● Chicken (4 ounces, skinless, size of a deck of cards): 35 grams

● Tuna (6 ounces, packed in water): 40 grams

● Fish (6 ounces of cod or salmon): 40 grams

● Lean red meat (4 ounces): 35 grams

● Lean pork (4 ounces): 35 grams

● Reduced-fat tofu (6 ounces): 30 grams

● Cottage cheese (1 cup, 1% or 2% fat): 28 grams

● Milk (1 cup of 1%, 2%, or fat-free): 8 grams

Remember, too, that your pre-workout shooter or post-workout recovery mix is going to contain 20 to 45 grams of protein per serving. (See "'Shot Clock' Pre- and Post-Exercise Nutrition" on pages 36 to 37.) If you have one or two shakes a day, along with some combination of poultry and fish for lunch and dinner and a breakfast that includes yogurt or egg whites, you'll easily meet your daily protein goal.

In addition to "eat a rainbow often," here's another rule of thumb regarding nutrition, specifically protein: "The less legs, the better." The fewer legs something has—or at least had when it was alive—the better its ratio of protein to healthy fat.

Fish, for instance, have no legs, and fish is a tremendously healthy source of protein, provided that it's not fried. Fish also provides omega-3 and omega-6 fatty acids, which promote cardiovascular health. Shellfish such as crab, lobster, shrimp, and prawns is the exception to "the less legs, the better" rule. Although they have many legs, they are better for you than red meat.

Chickens have two legs and also are a wonderful source of protein, provided the skin is removed and the meat is not fried.

Meat from four-legged creatures can be good, too, provided it's a lean cut—that's a key distinction. Red meat gets a bad rap, some of which is deserved since the heavily marbled meats are more tender and often have more flavor. But lean red meat is a tremendous source of important nutrients such as iron and phosphorus.

Pork, the so-called "other white meat," also gets a bad rap. It's usually fatty, but if you ask your butcher for a lean cut with little marbling, you'll have a tasty and nutritious protein.

Scouting Report: Fats

Strengths: Critical to good health and makeup of cell membranes. Fats release energy slowly, keeping the body sated and regulating blood sugar, and thus lowering glycemic response to other foods. Good fats provide powerful nutrients and antioxidants for cellular repair of the joints, organs, skin, and hair. Fats, especially those found in fish oil and flaxseed oil, also help with cognitive ability, mental clarity, and memory retention, and they have very strong anti-inflammatory properties.

Weaknesses: Not all fat is good—and saturated fats are very bad indeed. The difference in chemical structure between saturated and unsaturated fats produces significantly different effects on health. Saturated fats, which are usually found in meat and dairy foods and are solid at room temperature, raise serum cholesterol levels, clog arteries, and pose a risk to the heart.

At the same time, not all *un*saturated fats are healthy. Vegetable shortening is also unsatu-

rated, but it's unhealthy. That's because it contains trans fats, which raise bad (LDL) cholesterol but do not raise good (HDL) cholesterol. You may identify these trans fats on the label by looking for the words "partially hydrogenated soybean oil." This artery-clogging fat is found in processed foods such as cookies, crackers, pies, pastries, and margarine. It's also found in fried foods, especially those at fast-food restaurants, and in smaller quantities in meat and some dairy products. As of January 1, 2006, food manufacturers must list on their labels the amount of trans fat; some manufacturers have done so for more than a year. Even snack foods labeled "low-fat" can contain too much trans fat, so be sure to consult the labels.

Ideal Players:

- Oils: Fish oil, high-lignan flaxseed oil, extra virgin olive oil, canola oil, Enova brand oil

- Vegetables: Avocados

- Seeds: Pumpkin, sunflower, flaxseeds

- Nuts: Almonds, cashews, pecans, macadamias, soy nuts, walnuts. (Almonds were found in a recent study by *Men's Health®* magazine to have the most nutritional value, followed by cashews, pecans, and macadamias.)

Bottom Line: Good fats, in moderation, are great for you.

One of the biggest health trends of the last 20 years has been the anti-fat movement. Everything had to be low-fat, preferably fat-

42

free. "You are what you eat," according to the popular saying, and if you ate fat, you were going to end up looking like the Stay Puft marshmallow man.

The best fats come out of nuts, fish oils, and seeds. Few foods have such an undeserved bad rap as nuts. As part of the anti-fat movement, people avoided them because they were high in fat. But nuts and seeds are a convenient source of protein and fiber, and they stick with you longer than many snacks, helping control blood sugar and appetite. A handful of nuts every day may lower the risk of heart ailments and Alzheimer's disease. Unsaturated fats do not raise cholesterol levels, and research indicates that they actually can reduce it when substituted for saturated fats. The best unsaturated fats, liquid at room temperature, are found in olive oil, canola oil, flaxseed oil, Enova brand oil, and fish oils.

Fish oils provide powerful omega-3 and omega-6 fatty acids, which have antioxidant properties and are essential for good cardiovascular health and mental clarity. These are found in salmon, mackerel, lake trout, herring, sardines, and some types of white fish. Swordfish and tuna contain fatty acids, though not as much as salmon. Fish is a tremendous source of protein, and it doesn't hit you with the saturated fats like some fatty meats do.

Everyone should have a bottle of high-lignan flaxseed oil and/or fish oil in the refrigerator. The body can convert flaxseed oil into omega-3 and omega-6 fatty acids, much like fish oil. A tablespoon or two a day—one in the morning and one in the evening—is all you need, and it can go into a shake or on top of oatmeal.

Olive oil is another excellent choice. It has great antioxidant properties, is good for cooking, and goes well with salads. Enova brand oil is new to the market and actually gets burned as energy. It's less likely to be stored as fat, and has half the saturated fat of canola oil.

Scouting Report: Trans Fats

Strengths: None, though food manufacturers love that it's so cheap and easy to create trans fat by adding hydrogen to vegetable oil—a process called hydrogenation. Hydrogenation increases the shelf life and flavor of the foods containing these fats.

Weaknesses: Trans fat raises the LDL cholesterol that increases the risk of heart disease. According to a 9-year study of 16,500 men published in the *American Journal of Clinical Nutrition,* researchers found that for every 2 percent increase in trans fat intake, men added one-third of an inch to their waists over the course of a year.

Ideal Players: None. Trans fat is found everywhere—in vegetable shortenings, some margarines, cookies, crackers, snack foods, and other foods made with or fried in partially hydrogenated oils.

Bottom Line: Try to avoid products containing trans fat.

CORE NUTRITION STRATEGY #4: STAY HYDRATED

We tend to take water for granted. It's readily available, but instead we hydrate with inferior beverages ranging from soda to coffee to alcohol. For all of the advances in technology, we still have not come up with something better than water. It's the perfect beverage.

If I said that you could do up to 25 percent more work or run 25 percent farther, you'd sprint through a wall to make that happen, right? Actually, it's much easier. Just drink enough water before, during, and after exercise. Drink a gallon of water a day. Drink 2 cups of water first thing in the morning. Take a gallon jug to work and drink all day. Keep a bottle in the car.

If you want to reduce calories quickly, cut them out of your drinks. If you replace soft drinks, juices, sports drinks, and beer with water, or try "fitness" or "flavored" waters, you'll cut down on calories and sugar. Without those calories for energy, your body will burn body fat and the higher-fiber carbs recommended by the Core Nutrition game plan for energy. You'll lose fat and probably weight, too. For convenience, buy a case of bottled water and keep the bottles nearby in the refrigerator. That way you're more likely to grab water instead of sugary drinks.

Water has a direct impact on the aging process. Because of dehydration, inactivity, and trauma from daily life, the connective tissues around our muscles and joints dry up over time, sort of like those chew toys for dogs that start out soft and pliable and end up stiff and brittle. Drinking lots of water prevents this process while improving your muscle tissue and flexibility.

As far as artificial sweeteners in soft drinks and other beverages go, recent research suggests that *modest* consumption of artificial sweeteners is a better alternative to high-fructose corn syrup and other sugars. Although I'm not a fan of diet soft drinks—it is better to drink water—diet soda is a much better choice than a regular soft drink that's loaded with sugar. (A typical can of "regular" soda has about 150 calories, all from sugar.)

Instead of coffee, consider a healthier alternative such as green, white, or black tea. All of these teas have protective antioxidant properties.

Proper hydration regulates appetite. A lot of times, people think they're hungry when they're really just thirsty. If you're trying to lose weight, have a glass of water before eating—it will help prevent you from overeating.

Always "think before you drink." Are you drinking to stay hydrated, or to produce a certain response? If you substitute water for coffee, soda, and alcohol, you'll have no problem drinking a gallon a day. Drink two glasses when you wake up, two glasses with every meal, and plenty of water before, during, and after working out. You won't miss the caffeine. The Core Nutrition game plan helps you regulate your blood sugar and maintain your energy level, so you won't feel quite the need to use caffeine as an artificial energy source.

Don't assume that sports drinks are an adequate substitute for water, especially in everyday life. In fact, most are loaded with a ton of high-glycemic carbohydrates that elevate blood sugar and ultimately contribute to body fat (though sports drinks are critical for serious endurance athletes and for other athletes who compete in prolonged, intense activity). One of the most exciting hydration products to hit the market is one of my company's sponsors, Amino Vital, which contains a combination of branched chain amino acids (BCAAs), arginine, and glutamine to support immune health, muscle recovery, and improve mental function.

Scouting Report: Wine

Strengths: Studies suggest that moderate consumption of red wine reduces the risk of cardiovascular disease. Resveratrol, an antioxidant, is found in high concentrations in red grape skins. Some people also find that red wine enhances their enjoyment of food, especially red meats.

Weaknesses: Besides the obvious dangers of excessive alcohol consumption, alcohol also impairs our deep REM (rapid eye movement) sleep, which is essential for positive hormone release, body repair, and quality restful sleep. Alcohol consists of empty calories and lessens immune function. It decreases performance, slows the recovery process, impairs judgment, causes dehydration, and, of course, is addictive.

Ideal Players: Pinot Noir, Beaujolais, Shiraz, Merlot, Cabernet Sauvignon. If you don't drink alcohol, consider adding grape juice or grape seed extract supplements to your diet, to obtain antioxidant properties similar to those found in resveratrol.

Bottom Line: Alcohol contains 7 empty calories per gram and should be consumed only in moderation. One glass of red wine, a few times per week, is an acceptable part of the Core Nutrition program. Always consume one glass of water for each alcoholic drink to prevent dehydration.

Chapter 4 Summary: A few simple nutritional strategies will make a dramatic impact on your health. Eat smaller portions more often, spread evenly across the day, containing a combination of lean protein, healthy fats, and less-processed carbohydrates. Your carbohydrate intake should be relative to your activity level. Eat "glycemically correct" carbs, high in color and fiber—the less processed, the better. Drink plenty of water, and add a pre-workout shooter or post-workout recovery mix to your routine.

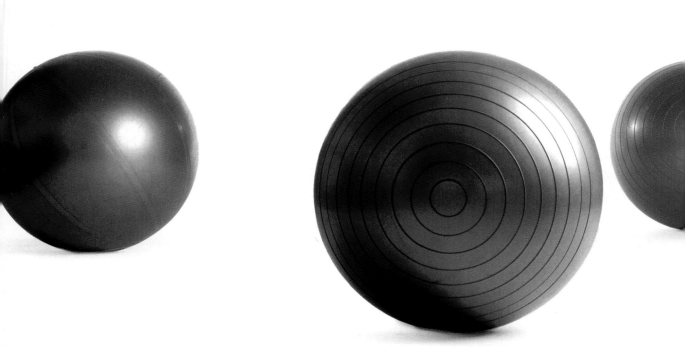

CHAPTER 5

GAME PLAN

n order to eat properly, you need to forget the traditional concept of the word *diet*. The connotation is negative—the first three letters are d-i-e—and diets are viewed as quick-fix, temporary solutions. From this point forward, you will have to make a conscious decision every time you eat something. Turn off your bad-habit autopilot and ask yourself, "Will this help me achieve my goals, or sabotage them?"

Start viewing your nutrition program as a game plan for your long-term health and productivity. It's a vital, core strategy for the rest of your life. Otherwise you take a reactive approach to eating, consuming whatever is out there, with little thought to how it affects you, in terms of both energy production and long-term health.

As with everything else in this book, I want you to be proactive about your diet. I recommend that you take 90 minutes each Saturday or Sunday to plan, shop, and prepare menus of meals for an entire week. It's easy and fun—and it saves money and time.

The problem with many diet plans is that they make you go cold turkey. *We're* not going to do that. Instead, let's take a more realistic approach.

CREATING THE HOME FIELD ADVANTAGE

Let's start in your kitchen. Think of yourself as the general manager of a sports team. In pro

CORE NUTRITION: 3 WEEKS TO RESHAPE YOUR LIFE

Week One: "Training Camp, 4 on 4"

We're going to stock the pantry, refrigerator, and freezer properly. We're going to eat four meals a day—4 days a week. The other 3 days? Try to do the same, but don't worry if you don't quite make it.

Week Two: "Preseason, 5 on 5"

Now we're going to eat five meals a day—5 days a week. Again, don't worry about the other 2 days.

Week Three: "Regular Season (and beyond), 6 on 6"

We're going to eat six meals a day, 6 days a week. Use the other day to eat what you like.

sports, the "GM" must work within constraints. He has a set budget. Perhaps there's some dead weight on the roster in the form of long-term, guaranteed contracts of players now injured or ineffective. No matter how hard the GM tries, he cannot dump those contracts on someone else.

Many people approach the assembly of their pantries and refrigerators the same way, even though they're not bound by any constraints. There's plenty of dead weight—both the junk in the pantry and the fat it has heaped on their bodies—but still, people continue to purchase more unhealthy food. They're like general managers that keep acquiring underachieving, expensive players that keep the team from winning.

If you look inside your pantry and refrigerator and see foods with little nutritional value, chances are you're not going to like what you see in the mirror either. How we look is a direct reflection of how we fuel our bodies and the amount of physical activity we engage in.

Embarking on a new nutrition program is im-

possible if your kitchen is filled with temptation. In order to eat properly, you must control the environment. I cannot stress enough how much our environment supports our habits, especially at home. It's more challenging to eat right when out of the house, especially while traveling. So at least give yourself a home field advantage by stocking your kitchen properly. If there's nothing bad in the house to eat, chances are you're going to eat properly.

We're going to "draft" a new team of good foods. But first, let's cut all of those bad players from our roster. Unlike the general manager, we're not stuck with anything. Take a trash can and go into the pantry. Toss away all those processed foods, such as cookies, crackers, snack chips, white pastas and rice, cake mixes, candy, creamy soups, sugary cereals, and soda. Open the refrigerator and discard beer, whole milk, creamy side dishes and casseroles, ice cream, fatty meats, white bread—anything that's not a high-performance food.

Wow, look at all that space you have! Now it's

time to go to the grocery store and draft a new team of players. Don't worry if you don't know where to find them, even if you've been shopping in the same place for years. We tend to be creatures of habit, rolling down the aisles on autopilot, grabbing the same foods we've eaten forever. But if you take just a moment and consider some healthier alternatives, many of which taste better, you can change your life. You'll look and feel better, have more energy, and live longer.

As you look inside that empty kitchen, you might wonder if there are any foods left out there. In fact, there are dozens. On page 50 is a list of foods we're going to obtain. I recommend that you photocopy the list and keep it in the glove compartment of your car.

THE DRAFT: LET'S GO SHOPPING

Now that you have your Core Nutrition strategies in place, we are going to arm you with a Core Nutrition shopping list and a map of the Core grocery store for recruiting the right players.

Before we go, it's important for you to understand how to get around the field—and manage to stay in bounds. We also have provided complete scouting reports for each department and the right shopping aisles. Fuel up before you go; it's never a good idea to shop hungry.

As you work through the grocery store, stay along the perimeter. Virtually everything you need is along the outer aisles, such as produce, fish, meat, and dairy products. Instead of going down every aisle, glance at the overhead signs to locate healthy items such as canned tuna fish, beans, frozen fruits, vegetables, protein, oatmeal, and olive oil. Leave the cart at one end and walk down the aisle. That way you avoid being tempted by cake mixes, cookies, chips, and soft drinks. And, as a bonus, you'll save time.

Most of us learn about foods from the worst possible places—the media, and, more specifically, advertisers. Much of what we hear from these sources isn't accurate, and what is accurate is at best incomplete. You have to fill in the blanks. Examine labels for content, especially the amounts of proteins, fats, and carbs contained. If you're good with numbers, try to calculate the percentages of each in the food. Look at the line that tells you how many grams of sugar are in the product, then look at the list of ingredients to see what kind of sugar it is. I've already explained that high-fructose corn syrup (or HFCS) is to be avoided. The same goes for trans fats.

All this reading and calculating might take a few extra minutes at first, but pretty soon you'll be able to cruise through the aisles—maybe even faster than before.

Though I use the term *supermarket,* I recognize that many people shop at warehouse stores. At one time, warehouse stores had a reputation for selling products only in quantities big enough to last a year or more. They still tend to sell in larger sizes than supermarkets do, but so what? Chances are that buying bigger sizes of Core Nutrition staples will save you money. You'll

(continued on page 52)

CORE GROCERY LIST

GENERAL SHOPPING TIPS:

● Stay focused. ● Avoid products at the heads of the aisles.
● Watch out at the checkout! ● Explore one new healthy food with each shopping trip.

BAKERY
100% whole wheat bread
(look for fiber)
Pumpernickel bread/products
Sourdough bread/products

CEREAL AISLE
Bran cereal
Kashi cereal (my personal favorite)

CANNED FOODS
Black beans
Fruit, packaged with no sugar added
Kidney beans
Navy beans
Pinto beans
Tuna, water-packed

DELI SECTION
TIP: Avoid deli salads and fried foods.
Deli meats, lean and reduced-fat
(turkey, chicken, roast beef, ham)
Hummus
Rotisserie chicken (remove skin
and pat down chicken)

MEAT & SEAFOOD AISLES
Chicken, skinless, white meat
Ground beef, 97% fat-free
Red meat and pork, lean
Salmon and other fish
Turkey, white meat

DAIRY SECTION
TIP: Avoid whole-milk products.
Cheese, reduced-fat
Cottage cheese, 2%, 1%, or fat-free

Juices, 100% juice, no sugar added
Milk, 1% or fat-free
Yogurt, low-fat, low-sugar

FROZEN FOODS
Fruits
Ice cream, low-fat, low-sugar
Juices, 100% juice, no sugar added
Kashi waffles
Soy yogurt or ice cream
Vegetables

BAKING, SNACK, AND CONDIMENT AISLES
Almonds
Canola oil
Enova oil
High-protein meal-replacement bars
Mustard
Olive oil
Peanut butter, natural
Peanuts
Salad dressing, low-fat
Sunflower seeds
Vinegar, balsamic or red wine
(for salads)

PRODUCE SECTION
TIPS: Stock it up!
Cut and package produce to eat later.
Apples, red or green
Apricots
Bananas
Blueberries
Broccoli

Carrots
Cauliflower
Cucumber
Edamame
Grapefruit
Grapes, red
Green beans
Kiwifruit
Oranges
Pears
Romaine lettuce
Spinach
Strawberries
Sweet potatoes
Tofu
Tomatoes

PHARMACY
Antioxidant complex
Calcium (for women)
Fish oil/omega-3 capsules (Udo's
Choice Blend is one good brand)
Multivitamin
Vitamin C (500 mg)
Vitamin E (400 IU)
Whey protein powder

BEVERAGE AISLES
Coffee, regular and decaf
Dry beverages
(such as Crystal Light)
Juices, 100% juice, no sugar added
Tea, green, white, and black
Water, bottled
Wine, red

SERVING SIZES
Vegetables: 1 cup raw vegetables, ½ cup cooked vegetables, ¾ cup vegetable juice, ½ cup cooked dry beans
Fruits: 1 medium-size fruit (1 medium apple or 1 medium pear), ½ cup canned or chopped fruit, or ¾ cup fruit juice
Breads and Cereals: 1 slice of bread, ⅔ cup ready-to-eat cereal, ½ cup cooked rice or pasta
Protein: 4 oz meat (the size of the palm of your hand), handful of nuts, 2 Tbsp peanut butter
Fats: 1 Tbsp olive oil, 1 Tbsp Enova oil, 1 Tbsp flaxseed oil, 1 Tbsp fish oil
Dairy: 1 cup milk, 1 cup cottage cheese, 1 oz or slice of cheese

CORE GROCERY STORE DIAGRAM

Stay along the perimeter of the store. Avoid the middle aisles, except for the occasional healthy item.

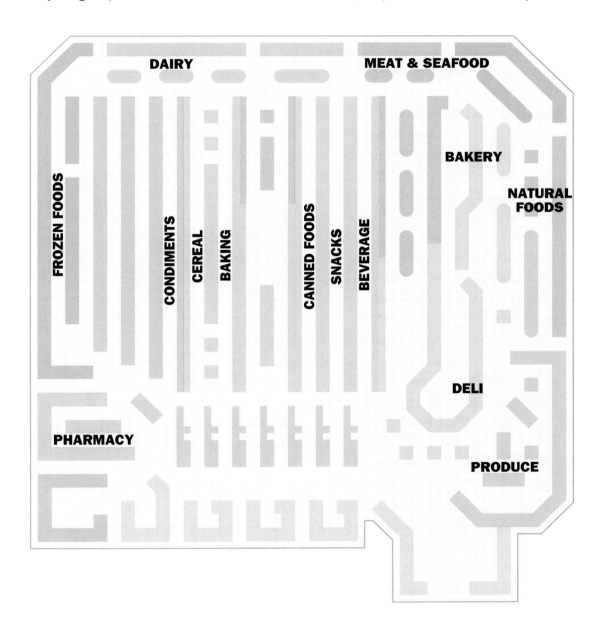

also save time since you can freeze what you don't use.

Now, let's go aisle by aisle through the supermarket and fill your grocery cart with high-quality Core foods. We've provided a scouting report for each area. Now it's time to go shopping.

Scouting Report: Dairy

Strengths: Dairy products are good sources of calcium, which supports bones. New research suggests that calcium intake may help lower body fat.

Weaknesses: Dairy products can add unnecessary calories to a meal. They often can be high in fat.

Ideal/Undervalued Players: Fat-free or 1% milk; reduced-fat cheese, cottage cheese, and cream cheese; fat-free or low-fat *plain* yogurt.

Pretenders: Low-fat and fat-free flavored yogurt often is loaded with empty calories in the form of sugar, which will send your blood sugar level soaring.

Bottom Line: Dairy products, in moderation, are good sources of calcium.

Scouting Report: Produce

Strengths: It's hard to go wrong in this section of the store. Since you want to "eat a rainbow often," you should fill up a good chunk of your cart right here. Fruit and vegetable platters are healthy alternatives to chips and dips to serve at parties. Prepackaged salads often can be found in the deli section. Garden salads are fine, provided that the dressing is on the side. Go easy on the croutons. As always, the more color, the better.

Salads with leafy spinach and romaine lettuce tend to be more colorful and nutrient-dense than those made predominantly with iceberg lettuce.

Weaknesses: None. This is the healthiest part of the supermarket.

Ideal Players: Foods rich in color and anti-oxidant properties, such as tomatoes, blueberries, spinach, asparagus, pomegranates, and broccoli. Salads with plenty of spinach and tomatoes are also terrific.

Undervalued Prospects: Just about any colorful, fiber-rich vegetable is undervalued. Soybeans are another power food. They're rich in nutrients and high in protein.

Pretenders: Dried fruits and trail mixes. They're calorie-dense and too heavy in sugar. Iceberg lettuce has little nutrient value.

Bottom Line: When choosing fruits and vegetables, fresh is the best way to go. Frozen fruit and veggies are preferable to canned goods, since nutrients are lost in the canning process.

Scouting Report: Deli

Strengths: Lean meat is a rich and convenient source of protein.

Weaknesses: Cheese is tempting for many people. When you eat cheese, do so in moderation—ideally, treat it as a garnish.

Ideal Players: Ninety-seven-percent fat-free, deli-sliced meats, and reduced-fat, deli-sliced cheeses. Generally speaking, softer cheeses have lower fat content, whereas hard cheese usually contains more of the bad saturated fats. But eat it only in moderation.

Undervalued Prospects: Rotisserie chicken is one of my favorites. It's flavorful, it's precooked, and it provides several meals out of a single chicken at an affordable price. The key is to drain the fat, remove the fatty skin, and pat the bird down with a paper towel.

Pretenders: Pasta salads, potato salad, and other creamy side dishes.

Bottom Line: You always want to go for the leanest cuts of meat and cheese possible. When selecting turkey, ham, and chicken, go for a brand that's at least 97 percent fat-free.

Scouting Report: Bread and Baked Goods

Strengths: This is an area where we may find some great low-glycemic, high-fiber carbohydrates.

Weaknesses: Avoid white, buttermilk, or split-top "wheat" breads; they have too much enriched flour (the stuff that's been heavily processed). Be on the lookout for high-fructose corn syrup; it even appears in bread. Bagels and English muffins should be eaten only in the morning and with the proper toppings (natural peanut butter, light cream cheese, and so forth). As for tortillas, go for the whole wheat, low-carb version.

Ideal Players: Tough to draft an ideal player here. If you eat bread, look for "stone-ground" or "crushed wheat." Whole wheat breads marketed as "light" generally tend to come in thinner slices, which is another way to keep from overdoing it on breads.

Undervalued Prospects: Rye, pumpernickel, and most types of sourdough typically fall in a lower range on the glycemic index than whole wheat bread. This can be an advantage in controlling blood sugar and energy. Whole wheat, however, can have more fiber than the other breads. Judging solely by glycemic rating, rye, pumpernickel, and sourdough might be superior, but because of its fiber content, whole wheat bread is the winner.

Pretenders: White breads, along with cake mixes, muffins, and brownies—pretty much the entire baked goods aisle.

Bottom Line: When choosing breads, opt for choices such as pumpernickel, rye, sourdough, or whole wheat, which have not been heavily processed. Don't be fooled by loaves of brown bread labeled as "wheat." If it's not made with whole wheat flour, it's just white bread dyed to look like something more nutritious.

Scouting Report: Condiments, Jellies, and Spices

Strengths: Condiments don't add much nutritional value, but small quantities make food tasty, ensuring that you'll stay with the program.

Weaknesses: Condiment labeling can be deceiving. Salad dressings are notoriously confusing. One manufacturer's "low-fat" might be comparable to the standard brand of another company. Whatever you choose, go easy on the dressing. It also pays to eyeball the jelly and jam labels. The lower the sugar content, the better. Straight fruit spreads (as opposed to preserves) are preferable.

Ideal Players: Hummus (pronounced "HUM-iss") is an exotic blend of lemon, chickpeas, garlic, sesame puree, and olive oil that contains no saturated fat, cholesterol, or sugar. It also contains protein and fiber. Spices such as oregano and parsley are a great way to get flavor without adding lots of calories.

Replace butter with a lower-calorie substitute such as I Can't Believe It's Not Butter! Light. Sprays are preferable to tub margarines, since there's a tendency to go overboard with spreads. You get better coverage and use less with the spray. Olive oil or Pam cooking spray, made from canola oil, is ideal for cooking.

Undervalued Prospects: Mustard, hummus, salsa, and horseradish are better alternatives to mayonnaise. Olive oil and balsamic vinegar are preferable to salad dressing. Extra virgin olive oil is best; it's produced from the first pressing of olives and has less than 1 percent acidity.

Peanut butter gets a bad rap. *Natural* peanut butter is better than run-of-the-mill creamy brands. Pour off about half of the oil floating at the top of natural peanut butter, and mix up the rest. If you must go with a standard peanut butter, be careful with the reduced-fat products. Manufacturers tend to pour in the high-fructose corn syrup.

Replace sugar with Splenda, a no-calorie sweetener that is made, according to its Web site, "through a patented process that starts with sugar and converts it to a no-calorie, non-carbohydrate sweetener."

Pretenders: Sugar, butter, mayonnaise, anything with high-fructose corn syrup.

Bottom Line: Spend some time reading the labels in this aisle. Whether it's salad dressing, barbecue sauce, ketchup, or mayonnaise, it's important to examine the grams of fat and sugar and the number of calories per serving. High-fructose corn syrup rears its ugly head often in this area, so if you are going to use condiments that contain it, do so in moderation, and pay attention to actual serving sizes.

Scouting Report: Cereals and Breakfast Foods

Strengths: With breakfast being the most important meal of the day, this aisle provides the quickest and easiest options.

Weaknesses: Besides being ridiculously expensive, many cereals provide only modest nutritional value. Too often, they're loaded with sugar and calories.

Ideal Players: The 5-minute version of old-fashioned Quaker Oats has been around forever but is still arguably the best cereal option. The 1-minute version and low-sugar prepackaged oatmeal products are more processed, but they still make a decent choice. The original Cheerios also are a good choice since they, too, are made from oats. Avoid the sugary versions of Cheerios. Lean breakfast meats and low-fat, low-sugar yogurts are also great choices.

Undervalued Prospects: Kashi's breakfast cereals, their flavored instant oatmeal, and their frozen waffles are high in fiber and an excellent breakfast choice. Egg whites or similar substitutes are preferable to eggs. For those times when you do bake, consider replacing eggs partially or fully with egg whites. (Two egg whites are equivalent to one egg.) Again, make the best choice possible, even if you're eating cake.

Pretenders: Sugary cereals, French toast, doughnuts, pastries, most waffles and pancakes, sugary fruit drinks.

Bottom Line: It's important to get the day started right. Rethink that big breakfast. For instance, pancakes are permissible as long as you don't make a complete meal out of them. There's nothing wrong with having one pancake with, say, an egg-white omelet. Use I Can't Believe It's Not Butter! spray instead of butter on your pancake. Use syrup sparingly and look for brands with little or no sugar. Not surprisingly, syrup often is loaded with high-fructose corn syrup.

Scouting Report: Fish and Meat

Strengths: Fish and meat are tremendous sources of protein, the building blocks of muscle.

Weaknesses: Some cuts of meat tend to be heavily marbled with those dangerous saturated animal fats.

Ideal Players: Salmon is one of the best power foods. Besides being a better source of protein than most meats, it's loaded with omega-3 fatty acids, which have heart disease–reducing properties. Not only that, but many people also find salmon more flavorful than other fish.

Undervalued Prospects: Contrary to popular belief, lean red meat is great for you. Lean cuts are high in protein, low in fat, and great sources of iron and phosphorus. Red meat should be consumed in moderation, but there's no reason to eliminate it from your diet.

A good strategy is to select cuts made from the animal's muscles of locomotion. Top and bottom round are lean cuts, since they come from the rear legs. They're named for the round bone of the femur. Flank cuts also are very lean, and cube steak is very lean. Avoid fattier, more marbled cuts such as strips, fillets, and T-bones. Lean pork is also a terrific choice, especially when grilled, or Shake 'n Baked.

Canned tuna fish is an excellent source of protein; just make sure it's canned in water, not vegetable oil.

Pretenders: Fatty meat, battered or breaded fish, creamy seafood salads.

Bottom Line: Remember the rule: The less legs, the better. It's tough to go wrong with fish, though it should be baked, grilled, or broiled— never fried or breaded. After fish, chicken and other types of poultry have the fewest legs. Cornish game hens are a good alternative, though like chicken they should be stripped of skin. As with fish, poultry never should be fried or breaded.

Scouting Report: Pasta and Side Dishes

Strengths: Not many. A small, tennis-ball-size serving of pasta—preferably whole wheat or vegetable pasta—is acceptable. Go with low-sugar, meatless pasta sauce. Add lycopene-rich tomato paste and a little olive oil, or make your own sauce, adding extra-lean ground beef or turkey.

Weaknesses: Pasta is high-glycemic, and it has a very high glycemic load, meaning that a small portion can send blood sugar levels soaring.

Ideal Players: Whole wheat pasta in small quantities. When choosing rice, go with brown rice, wild rice, and seven-grain rice pilaf. Brown rice has more fiber than white rice, because it's less processed.

Undervalued Prospects: A better alternative to rice is couscous. Pronounced "koos-koos," it's a staple of North African cooking and is made from durum wheat, the ideal pasta wheat because of its high protein content.

Pretenders: Overcooked pastas, white pastas, white rice.

Bottom Line: The key to pasta and rice is to go whole grain, don't cook them very long, and look at them as a side dish, not as an entire meal.

Scouting Report: Snacks

Strengths: Low-glycemic, nutrient-dense snacks are a quick and easy way to control midafternoon hunger pangs.

Weaknesses: If you have a hankering for something sweet, try a low-sugar frozen-fruit bar. If you're a chocoholic, go with a fat-free Fudgsicle, which is low in sugar and has just 60 calories. When choosing ice cream or frozen yogurt, look for brands that are low in fat and sugar. (A fat-free brand might be heavy in high-fructose corn syrup.) Buy small containers of ice cream, since studies suggest that the larger the container, the larger the serving a person will take.

Ideal Players: Almonds; sunflower seeds; beef jerky; low-fat yogurt with no sugar added (add in fiber with oats, nuts, seeds, or a teaspoon of flaxseed or fish oil); fruits; veggies; good protein snack bars (see below).

Undervalued Prospects: Protein bars can be a great late-afternoon "meal." Unfortunately, many of these so-called meal-replacement bars have the same nutritional value as candy bars. Ideally, look for a snack bar that has a carbs-to-protein ratio of no more than 2:1—generally, the more protein, the better. So if a bar has 30 grams of carbs, it should have at least 15 grams of protein. Many new products have a higher ratio of protein, such as 1:2, meaning 15 grams of carbs and 30 grams of protein.

Pretenders: Granola bars, cereal bars, trail mixes, dried fruit, high-sugar yogurts, all other sugary products, salted and sugary nuts, and high-fat, low nutrient-value crackers, etc. This last option tends to be highly processed, calorie-dense, and high in sugar and/or bad fats.

Bottom Line: Individual preferences vary widely when it comes to meal-replacement bars. If you've had bad experiences with them in the past, give them another chance.

Scouting Report: Beverages

Strengths: Proper hydration is essential for health.

Weaknesses: For many people, life is impossible without coffee. The Core Performance Essentials program, which emphasizes proper sleep and meal timing, should wean you away from caffeine addiction. When you do drink coffee, don't go "grande," and don't overdo the cream and sugar. Try Splenda instead.

If you must have soft drinks, go with a diet beverage. I don't advocate diet soft drinks by any means—giving up soft drinks might be the easiest way for you to get more water—but if you must have them, find a diet brand you like. These will keep you hydrated, but water still is the best choice.

Ideal Players: Water is *the* ideal beverage. Pick up a case of 12- or 16-ounce bottles to take to work, to the gym, or in your car when you're out running errands. If you live in an area with poor-quality water, buy gallon jugs of distilled water, or use a water filtration system.

Undervalued Prospects: Green or white tea is a great substitute for coffee. I call them "power drinks," since they're natural sources of antioxidants. If you must have sugar with your coffee or tea, go with Splenda. Fat-free milk or 1% is better than whole or 2%. This rule applies to all dairy products.

Be careful when choosing fruit juices or fruit drinks—they often have too much sugar and high-fructose corn syrup. Always look for alternatives that are 100 percent fruit juice. Most juice can be diluted further with water, which lowers its glycemic load per ounce. You'll also get more out of it, which is a good thing since juice, like cereal, is usually overpriced.

Pretenders: Soda and fruit drinks. Choose sports drinks for the right reason; make sure they don't contain high-fructose corn syrup, a standard ingredient in many sport and fruit drinks. Avoid the self-serve soda fountains at restaurants unless you're going for the water, which, incidentally, is highly filtered and purified.

Bottom Line: Unless you're a serious endurance athlete or strength training, someone who's involved in running, biking, or other strenuous activities for long periods of time, you probably don't need anything more than water. You definitely don't need sports drinks for routine refreshment around the house or at work. (Remember: Think before you drink. Avoid drinking empty calories.)

Chapter 5 Summary: We have prepared ourselves for success by rewiring our mindset and creating powerful changes in our environment. Unlike traditional, quick-fix diet plans, the Core Nutrition program is a long-term plan to fuel your body for maximum daily energy and long-term success. Instead of requiring you to go cold turkey, this program includes a 3-week indoctrination program. Each meal should consist of a lean protein source along with low-to-midglycemic, colorful, and fiber-rich carbohydrates, and healthy fats in moderation. Always strive to make the best choice possible.

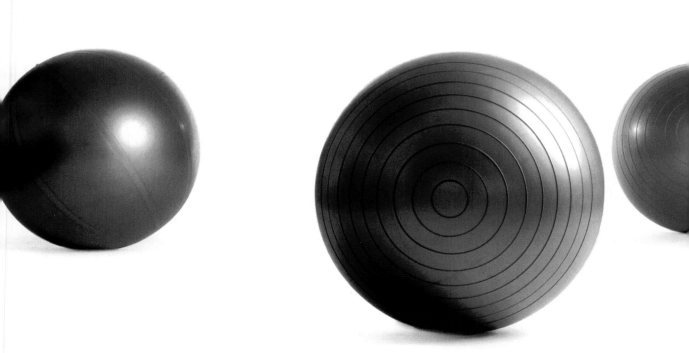

WINNING AT HOME

Planning is the key to eating properly, and in 3 weeks you're going to change the way you eat. In Week One, we'll do away with all of those bad foods and start eating four quality meals a day, 4 days a week. We'll stock our kitchen and office, as we will discuss in this chapter. In Week Two, we'll build upon that momentum and go for five good meals a day, 5 days a week.

Now that we have these empowering foods around, it's tough to make a bad decision. Not only that, but we also feel great about the decisions we're making because we can see the benefit of all this effort. We're transforming our bodies and producing more energy. We're benefiting from these new routines.

By Week Three, we will have established habits for life. We have the energy and a plan to sustain it regardless of what curveballs get thrown at us in the Game of Life.

If you fail nutritionally, it's almost certainly due to a lack of planning. So, instead of embarking on a mere diet, we're going to make a lifestyle change to produce more energy and protect the immune system. This will be the foundation for everything we do. We now have home field advantage.

You don't have to be perfect. Remember,

you're approaching this like an athlete, and even the best athletes do not create perfect results. A great basketball player shoots 50 percent from the field. The best baseball players produce hits just 30 percent of the time. From time to time, you will fall off this plan, and that's okay. But just jump right back on; you only fail if you give up.

One of the key components to my work with professional athletes is what I call "motivation through education." I could just tell you to consume the foods listed above and hope you'll follow my suggestions. But you'll be more mo-tivated once you understand *why* we're eating this way, and you'll know that you can pull it off because we have given you simple strategies for success.

Eating well, like working out properly, is a matter of understanding a few concepts, which we have shared with you, and creating a great plan to implement them. If you have the proper nutrition system in place, you'll find that eating healthfully is less stressful, less expensive, and more enjoyable.

I'll show you how to get the most nutrients out of your foods and how to create a champi-

SUNDAY—THE "OFF" DAY

Schedule one day a week that you call your "off" day from training and nutrition. Since Sunday is an off day from the Core Workout, feel free to take the day off nutritionally as well. This doesn't mean that you should in-hale an entire lasagna with a six-pack and a side of German chocolate cake, but it's okay to treat yourself. You've worked hard all week and you deserve to relax. Not only that, but having that treat provides a psycho-logical benefit: It helps you realize that you're not completely depriving yourself of foods you enjoy, even if they aren't particularly good for you.

It's unrealistic to think that you're going to eat nothing but healthy foods 42 times a week (six meals a day for 7 days). So take Sundays off. Remember, even elite pros who train at Athletes' Performance allow them-selves an occasional indulgence.

Don't be surprised, however, if many of those foods you used to love no longer seem appealing. You'll find that they no longer make you feel good, even in the short term. Once you've made this connection, feeling the response from your body, that's when you know you've taken this program to a higher level.

Sunday should also be your day to plan the week ahead. Shop, prepare meals, and create a game plan for the upcoming week's meals and snacks. Write a list of the available ingredients that you can build meals around. Use Sunday to pat yourself on the back for the successful regeneration.

onship meal plan that includes the proper amount of proteins, carbs, fats, fiber, vitamins, and minerals. You'll see how to combine foods for a powerful nutritional value and to maximize energy.

CORE MEAL #1:
MAKE BREAKFAST THE MOST IMPORTANT MEAL OF THE DAY

Think of breakfast as "break-the-fast," which is exactly what you're doing. When you wake up in the morning, your body is in a fasted state. During sleep, it uses the available nutrients for repair and energy, and by the time you wake up, there's usually nothing left. Your tank is empty, and the body will turn to your lean muscle stores for energy.

By skipping breakfast, as many people do, you actually increase the risk of obesity. In fact, researchers at the University of Massachusetts found that not eating breakfast increases the risk of obesity by 450 percent! Eating breakfast *away* from home increased the risk 137 percent, no doubt because you're less likely to eat immediately and less likely to eat healthfully.

Since we'll have a nutrient-dense, slow-releasing snack before bedtime, we're going to give the body what it wants so that it doesn't tap into its lean muscle stores. Breakfast is going to ensure that your body

doesn't consume its muscle for food, a process known as *catabolism.* Breakfast also increases metabolism, fuels the brain, and provides energy.

It's important that breakfast include protein, fiber-rich carbohydrates, *and* good fats. Add a small glass of 100 percent fruit juice or a larger glass of diluted 100 percent fruit juice to make a complete breakfast. The key here is buying 100 percent fruit juice, which is much different than a "fruit drink" with real juice added. These fruit drinks are usually sweetened with high-fructose corn syrup.

Instead of drinking juice, why not try eating the original fruit with a glass of water? Consume an orange instead of juice. There's nothing wrong with OJ, of course, but remember that because it's already been processed for you, it's going to give you a higher glycemic response than the piece of fruit itself. Eating an orange also gives you the added fiber and nutrients. Let your body be the manufacturing plant, squeezing out all the nutrients that the orange has to offer.

Another good option is low-fat, low-sugar yogurt, which tastes better, sticks with you longer, and helps regulate blood sugar levels. It also can be a good source of protein and digestive enzymes. Add in some extra fiber, nuts, or flaxseeds. It's also tasty when mixed with oatmeal.

Top Power Breakfasts

"Breakfast Goulash"

$\frac{1}{2}$ cup uncooked oats

$1\frac{1}{2}$ scoops EAS whey protein powder

$\frac{1}{4}$ cup water

6 ounces low-fat, low-sugar blueberry yogurt

10 almonds

1 teaspoon flaxseed oil

Stir the oats and whey protein powder together dry. Add the water and stir wet. Add the yogurt, almonds, and flaxseed oil. Enjoy!

Makes 1 serving.

RECIPE NUTRIENT ANALYSIS (PER SERVING)
593 Calories (kcal), 40g Protein, 27% Calories from Protein, 51g Carbohydrates, 34% Calories from Carbohydrates, 25g Fat, 38% Calories from Fat, 3.5g Saturated Fat, 6g Total Dietary Fiber

"Hot Stuff"

1 packet Kashi low-sugar oatmeal

$\frac{2}{3}$ cup water

6 ounces Yoplait low-fat/low-sugar yogurt or unsweetened applesauce

3 capsules fish oil

Heat the oatmeal and water for 2 minutes. Add the yogurt or applesauce and the fish oil capsules. (Don't break the capsules open.) Serve with a bottle of water.

Makes 1 serving.

RECIPE NUTRIENT ANALYSIS (PER SERVING) (YOGURT VERSION)
244 Calories (kcal), 9g Protein, 16% Calories from Protein, 35g Carbohydrates, 60% Calories from Carbohydrates, 6g Fat, 24% Calories from Fat, 1g Saturated Fat, 3g Total Dietary Fiber

RECIPE NUTRIENT ANALYSIS (PER SERVING) (APPLESAUCE VERSION)
231 Calories (kcal), 4g Protein, 7% Calories from Protein, 40g Carbohydrates, 69% Calories from Carbohydrates, 6g Fat, 24% Calories from Fat, 1g Saturated Fat, 4g Total Dietary Fiber

Breakfast Bagel

1 egg

1 egg white

1 slice Canadian bacon

1 slice low-fat Cheddar cheese

1 pumpernickel, rye, or whole wheat bagel

In a small bowl, whisk the egg and egg white together. Pour into a microwave-safe bowl that is about the size of a bagel, and microwave on high power for 60 to 70 seconds. Top the egg mixture with the Canadian bacon and cheese. Microwave for another 50 to 60 seconds. Meanwhile, slice the bagel in half and toast it. Turn the egg mixture onto 1 bagel half, and top with the other half.

Makes 1 serving.

RECIPE NUTRIENT ANALYSIS (PER SERVING)
511 Calories (kcal), 42g Protein, 33% Calories from Protein, 63g Carbohydrates, 50% Calories from Carbohydrates, 10g Fat, 17% Calories from Fat, 3g Saturated Fat, 4g Total Dietary Fiber

CORE MEALS #2 AND #3: FOR LUNCH AND DINNER, THINK COMBO

When planning lunch and dinner, it's vital to include a combination of lean protein and some brightly colored carbs that are rich in fiber. You want to have some good fat, too, from olive oil, fish, nuts, or seeds. The foods will balance each other to produce maximum energy, build lean mass, and regulate your blood sugar level.

We have a tendency in our busy culture to skip lunch or eat something on the run that offers poor nutritional value, but you should take the time to pack your lunch the night before. Always take a designated time to eat lunch and relax for a few minutes, even if you get stuck in the office. Sit down and eat lunch away from your desk if possible. It helps break up the day and gets you refreshed to have a more productive afternoon. Don't wait until you are starving to eat. Be more proactive and control your hunger; don't let it control you.

When planning dinners, consider everyone's schedules; it's important information that will help you plan accordingly. Are you preparing dinner for one, two, or more, or do you need to prepare enough for everyone and set some aside for when they actually arrive? Good scheduling will also help you block out time to get everyone around one table, so that you can nourish your relationships while you nourish your body.

Top Power Assemblies for Lunch or Dinner

Surprisingly Simple Salmon

1 tablespoon olive oil

Lawry's fish seasoning to taste

1 5-ounce salmon fillet

1 10-ounce bag of fresh baby spinach, prewashed

15 baby tomatoes

Add the olive oil to a medium pan and heat on medium-high. Sprinkle the seasoning on both sides of the salmon and add the salmon to the pan. Pan-sear for 3 to 6 minutes on each side. Add the spinach and tomatoes. Cover and cook for 2 minutes, or until the fish is opaque and the spinach is wilted. Take the salmon out of the pan and pat it with a paper towel. Put the salmon in the center of a plate and surround it with the cooked vegetables.

Makes 1 serving.

RECIPE NUTRIENT ANALYSIS (PER SERVING)
504 Calories (kcal), 46g Protein, 36% Calories from Protein, 22g Carbohydrates, 17% Calories from Carbohydrates, 27g Fat, 47% Calories from Fat, 4g Saturated Fat, 10g Total Dietary Fiber

BBQ Salmon

2 4-ounce salmon fillets

6 tablespoons low-fat Catalina or French dressing

Salt and ground black pepper to taste

¼ cup low-fat Cheddar cheese

1 sourdough pita

Heat the grill to medium-high. Coat the shiny side of a large piece of aluminum foil with cooking spray. Place it shiny side up on the grill rack.

Place the fillets on the foil and coat each one with 3 tablespoons of the dressing. Sprinkle the top of each fillet with salt and pepper, then fold the foil up only around the edges so that the fish simmers in its own juice while exposed.

Continue grilling the salmon for 12 to 20 minutes, or until white bubbles appear on the top of the salmon. (It should be flaky when done.) Remove the fish from the grill and serve.

It's delicious with steamed, frozen organic broccoli sprinkled with low-fat shredded cheese; tomato slices; and sourdough bread.

Makes 2 servings.

RECIPE NUTRIENT ANALYSIS (PER SERVING)
567 Calories (kcal), 54g Protein, 37% Calories from Protein, 53g Carbohydrates, 36% Calories from Carbohydrates, 17g Fat, 26% Calories from Fat, 3g Saturated Fat, 7g Total Dietary Fiber

Spinach Salad

You can purchase precooked chicken breasts in most supermarkets, or cook them yourself as directed here.

2 5-ounce precooked chicken breasts, sliced or diced

1 10-ounce bag fresh spinach leaves

2 cups thinly sliced strawberries

¼ cup slivered almonds

6 ounces low-fat raspberry vinaigrette, such as Newman's Own

To cook the chicken: Preheat the oven to 400°F. Line a baking sheet or pie pan with aluminum foil coated with cooking spray. Place the chicken breast(s) on the foil. Season as desired—garlic powder, dried oregano, salt, and ground black pepper are good. Bake 10 to 15 minutes or until the chicken is no longer pink inside. Allow to cool before you slice or dice for the salad.

To assemble the salad: Place everything except the chicken in a large bowl and toss to coat. Split the salad onto two plates. Arrange the chicken slices or chunks on top of the salads.

Makes 2 servings.

RECIPE NUTRIENT ANALYSIS (PER SERVING)
336 Calories (kcal), 33g Protein, 38% Calories from Protein, 28g Carbohydrates, 33% Calories from Carbohydrates, 13g Fat, 34% Calories from Fat, 1g Saturated Fat, 6g Total Dietary Fiber

"I looked great for my wedding."

NAME: MATTHEW KEENER

AGE: 30

HOMETOWN: PHILADELPHIA

Medical school had taken its toll on Matthew Keener. A competitive rower, cyclist, and runner during his undergraduate years, he found it difficult to organize an exercise regimen around a grueling medical school schedule.

The long hours kept him from eating healthfully or regularly. He experienced wild fluctuations in energy levels. At one point, during a surgical rotation, he almost fell asleep at the operating table while watching a procedure.

When he began the Core program, he discovered that the nutrition philosophies meshed with what he was learning in school.

"I knew from studying the glycemic index that having three large meals and nothing in between would wreak havoc on me," he said. "Not only that, but it causes you to pack on the weight instead of building muscle or maintaining your existing lean mass."

Once a rock-solid, 6-foot-5, 185-pound triathlete, Keener had become a soft 190-pounder, literally a starving student. With his fiancée handling the bulk of their wedding preparations, he decided it was time to do some planning of his own to meet the demands of his busy schedule.

Keener set out time each week to assemble ready-to-go meals. He made sure he had plenty of meal-replacement drinks and bars on hand at all times. "The bars have been lifesavers," he says. "I can throw them in my white coat or backpack and no matter how busy I get, I can always eat one of those."

The program forced him to plot out his week. "If I knew I wasn't going to be near a gym for 2 days, I knew I could still use the physioball at home and do some Movement Prep." (To learn more, see part 3.) "It was just a matter of spending a half-hour to set the schedule for the week."

The Core Workout, along with better nutrition, gave Keener consistent energy and mental focus throughout the day. Core training also solved a nagging rotator cuff injury suffered during a skiing accident.

By the day of his wedding, August 21, 2004, Keener was a lean 205 pounds. "I looked great for my wedding," says Keener, who graduated from the University of Pittsburgh School of Medicine in 2005 and plans to pursue a career in psychiatry. "But more important, I've been able to keep that weight on and now have a program in place that will keep me on track no matter how busy I become as a doctor."

Shrimp and Asparagus

8 asparagus spears

2 lemons

10 ounces defrosted precooked shrimp
(see note)

1 teaspoon low-sodium seafood seasoning,
such as Lawry's

1 tablespoon extra virgin olive oil

Salt and ground black pepper to taste

Remove the tough bottoms of the asparagus stalks by holding them in both hands and bending. Discard the tough portions and chop each tender portion into three pieces. Set aside. Juice each lemon into separate containers and set these aside. Sprinkle the shrimp with the seafood seasoning and set aside. Heat a large sauté pan to medium-high. Add the olive oil and the reserved asparagus. Toss for about 2 minutes. Add the juice of 1 lemon, and toss in the pan for 1 more minute. Create a circle in the middle of the pan and add the shrimp. Toss the shrimp and asparagus together briefly, then cover and steam for 1 to 2 minutes, until the shrimp is heated through. Season with salt and pepper to taste. Add more lemon juice if desired.

Note: *To defrost shrimp safely, place it in the refrigerator overnight.*

Makes 1 serving.

RECIPE NUTRIENT ANALYSIS (PER SERVING)
399 Calories (kcal), 32g Protein, 33% Calories from Protein, 29g Carbohydrates, 30% Calories from Carbohydrates, 16g Fat, 37% Calories from Fat, 2g Saturated Fat, 2g Total Dietary Fiber

Taco Salad or Soft Tacos

In this recipe, you cook enough meat for 4 servings. You can serve them all at once, or refrigerate 3 servings' worth of cooked meat and leftover produce for later.

1 tablespoon extra virgin olive oil

1¼ pounds lean ground turkey

1 packet prepackaged taco seasoning

1 large tomato, diced

4 ounces low-fat shredded Cheddar cheese
(four 1-ounce servings)

1 large avocado, diced at serving time

8 ounces fat-free sour cream (four
2-ounce servings)

8 ounces salsa (four 2-ounce servings)

If making the salad:

4 heads romaine lettuce (1 head per serving)

1 15-ounce can black beans, drained and rinsed

1 10-ounce package defrosted frozen broccoli
florets

If making the tacos:

4 low-fat, high-fiber, low-carb 10" flour tortillas
(1 per serving)

1 head romaine lettuce (about 8 leaves,
shredded; optional)

To cook the turkey: Put the oil in a large sauté pan, heat over medium-high heat, and add the turkey, following the directions on the taco seasoning packet to cook and season the meat. When the turkey is no longer pink, remove it from the heat and set aside. If saving it for later, refrigerate immediately.

To make 1 serving of salad: Chop 1 head of

the lettuce and place it in a large salad bowl. Top with ¼ of the canned black beans, ¼ of the tomato, ¼ of the broccoli florets, and 1 ounce of the cheese. (To make 4 salads, quadruple these amounts.) Refrigerate until ready to serve. At serving time, add ¼ of the avocado to each salad, then spoon ¼ of the turkey meat over the top of each. Garnish each with 2 ounces of the sour cream and 2 ounces of salsa.

To make 1 taco: Microwave 1 soft tortilla on high power for 30 seconds or until soft enough to roll. Place the tortilla on a flat surface and spoon ¼ of the turkey meat down the center of the tortilla. Top with ¼ of the tomato, 2 shredded lettuce leaves (if desired), 1 ounce of shredded cheese, and ¼ of the diced avocado. (To make 4 tacos, quadruple these amounts.) Roll up each tortilla and serve each with 2 ounces of sour cream and 2 ounces of salsa.

Makes 4 taco salads or 4 soft tacos.

TACO SALAD RECIPE NUTRIENT ANALYSIS (PER SERVING)

576 Calories (kcal), 59g Protein, 41% Calories from Protein, 39g Carbohydrates, 27% Calories from Carbohydrates, 21g Fat, 33% Calories from Fat, 6g Saturated Fat, 11g Total Dietary Fiber

SOFT TACO RECIPE NUTRIENT ANALYSIS (PER SERVING)

716 Calories (kcal), 63g Protein, 35% Calories from Protein, 61g Carbohydrates, 34% Calories from Carbohydrates, 24g Fat, 30% Calories from Fat, 6g Saturated Fat, 13g Total Dietary Fiber

CORE SNACKS:
EAT BETWEEN PERIODS

If you've ever attended a sporting event, you've probably grazed throughout the game. After all,

3 hours is a long time to go without eating. Not wanting to miss any of the action, you wait until halftime or between periods to find a snack.

Though there are few healthy options available at the stadium, at least you're staying fueled. Ironically, people tend to nourish themselves more for spectator sports than they do for the Game of Life, where they endure long stretches of the workday with little fuel.

From a young age, many of us were taught to avoid eating between meals. We'll get fat and, at the very least, spoil our dinners. At least that's what a generation of moms led us to believe.

Actually, spoiling dinner is not such a bad thing if it means you won't overeat, as most people do. You need to keep your blood sugar levels consistent to minimize overeating. The only way to do this is to eat every 2½ to 3 hours.

Of course, we don't want to consume the equivalent of ballpark food. As with your meals, you want your snacks to include a combination of high-fiber carbohydrates, proteins, and fats. You could have a cup of low-fat cottage cheese or low-fat yogurt (with no added sugar). You could have a piece of fruit with natural peanut butter, and a handful of nuts. Beef jerky is a good snack. A little tuna or chicken combined with a fruit or vegetable also works.

For some people, there might be little difference between their meals and their snacks. Breakfasts, lunches, and dinners might be smaller than what you've traditionally eaten, since you are no longer trying to eat enough to curb your appetite for the next 6 to 12 hours.

Then again, the size of your meals might remain consistent, with your snacks being somewhat modest. That's okay, too, as long as snacks contain protein, high-fiber carbs, and good fats. For time and convenience, you might want to have a protein shake or a high-protein meal-replacement bar.

The challenge with meal-replacement bars is to find something that tastes good and is good for you. Look at the label carefully. Your goal is to find something with 15 to 30 grams of protein, 8 to 20 grams of carbs, and a few grams of fat. These include the EAS Myoplex Lite or Advantage bar and the Clif Bar line.

You have snacks or shakes built into your schedule three times a day. You might find the late-afternoon feeding the most important, since people tend to feel most sluggish at that time.

For your final snack at night, you'll want something that's going to stick with you, since it will be a long time before you eat again. Some chicken or fish left over from dinner would be a good snack; a protein shake or EAS ready-to-drink product would also work, as would a green apple with peanut butter. Whatever you choose, look for something with plenty of fiber.

So don't feel guilty about those between-meal snacks. In fact, look at them not as guilty pleasures but as essential components of a healthy lifestyle.

CORE SUPPLEMENTS

Walk into any health food store and you'll find a dizzying array of powders, capsules, and drinks that promise to transform your body. For simplicity, we're not going to bother with most of them in this book.

You already know that I recommend a pre-workout shooter or post-workout recovery mix, and shakes as snacks. It's also a good idea to take a multivitamin in the morning, along with an antioxidant complex, which is chock-full of vitamins and minerals.

If you're eating well and following this program, you can get by without antioxidant supplementation. But even elite athletes who come to Athletes' Performance and have their blood analyzed almost always are found to be deficient in some antioxidants. We immediately put them on supplements, and here's why: Whenever our bodies endure stress—whether from physical activity, sun damage, pollution, or the day-to-day demands of families and jobs—we suffer cellular damage. It's unavoidable. Those damaged cells are known as free radicals. We want to minimize their impact and get them out of our systems immediately.

Think of free radicals as hockey players fighting. Antioxidants are the referees that escort them to the penalty box. They maintain order among your cells and slow the aging process. They're critical to your immediate and long-term health. You can find a bottle of antioxidants at a health food store or supermarket for about $10. We recommend a product called Vitrin to our athletes—though it's more expensive than

THE DESK DRAWER CORE MVP

One of the biggest obstacles to eating right and maintaining optimal energy is dealing with the hunger pangs that hit throughout the day, especially in an office setting.

Well, no matter what our moms said, between-meal snacks, or "planned grazing," is the only way to properly fuel your body. This doesn't mean stuffing your face all day long, but instead it means planning what you graze on at specific points throughout the day. But who has time to go out and get something? Even the proactive people who bring their own lunches don't always have time to bring in snacks as well.

The last thing you want to do is resort to a vending machine, which is why I keep a desk drawer stocked with healthy food options. I have a box of oatmeal, tear-open packaged tuna fish, jerky, apples, oranges, and *healthy* snack bars. There's a jar of almonds, a loaf of whole wheat bread, condiments in one-serving packs, one-serving containers of sugar-free applesauce, plastic utensils, paper plates, and hand wipes. I have one of those mini-refrigerators near my desk and I keep it full of bottled water, fresh veggie snacks, fat-free yogurt with no sugar added, and ready-to-drink products.

Your "drawer" doesn't literally have to be in the office. It could be a container you keep in the car, or part of a diaper bag if you're a busy parent. This space has become the Most Valuable Player (MVP) of my nutrition program since it often saves me from making bad nutritional choices or trying to get through an afternoon hungry.

No matter how busy I am—and like many people, I find there are times when I can't leave my desk because of constant phone calls, meetings, and e-mails—I know that I'll be okay because of the trusty drawer, which I restock periodically. It's not just for snacks; there are adequate supplies for breakfast or lunch if I need it.

Encourage your co-workers, employees, and boss to create their own MVP drawers. It will raise office productivity by keeping energy high and eliminating lengthy midafternoon breaks to hunt for snacks. You'll set an example, thus elevating others. Most important, it will keep everyone on track with a healthy nutritional program.

run-of-the-mill antioxidants, two Vitrin caplets contain 29 essential vitamins and minerals, plus the antioxidant equivalent of five servings of fruits and vegetables.

There's been a lot of concern in recent years about supplements, much of it well-deserved. There's stuff you can buy legally in a health food store that I strongly caution our athletes against taking, either because of anecdotal evidence that suggests it's harmful or because no long-term studies have been conducted on the effects. With this in mind, I recommend that you stick to the supplemental foods recommended in this book.

Chapter 6 Summary: To eat healthfully and consistently, start thinking of meals not as traditional, sit-down affairs involving intensive preparation but as simple, quick "meal assemblies" involving a lean protein source, color- and fiber-rich carbohydrates, and healthy fats.

CORE MEAL ASSEMBLY

By now, your shopping cart should be bulging with foods that taste great and have tremendous nutritional value. The biggest misperception about eating right is that your meals have to be bland and boring, with little flavor. Nothing could be further from the truth. By using just the items mentioned below—and in earlier chapters—you can produce dozens of rich, tasty meals.

I'm not suggesting that you give up your favorite recipes. Many people are talented in the kitchen, and one of the joys of life is sharing a leisurely meal with friends and family. But most of the time, we just want something quick and easy. We're in no mood to cook after work. Besides, there's often not enough time to prepare an elaborate meal, because of demanding schedules.

The key is to stop looking at food in terms of lengthy preparation and instead view it as meal "assembly." Take a lean protein source, some carbohydrates rich in color and fiber, and some nutritious fats and you've got a great meal. This process goes hand-in-

SERVING SIZE GUIDE

This list can serve as a basic guide when you're substituting one form of food for another. Remember that whole foods are always better for you than processed foods or juices, because your body has to work harder to digest them.

Vegetables: 1 cup raw veggies, ½ cup cooked veggies, ¾ cup vegetable juice, ½ cup cooked dry beans

Fruits: 1 medium-size fruit (1 medium apple or medium pear), ½ cup canned or chopped fruit, or ¾ cup fruit juice

Breads and Cereals: 1 slice of bread, ⅔ cup ready-to-eat cereal, ½ cup cooked rice or pasta

Protein: 4 ounces meat (the size of a deck of cards), a handful of nuts, 2 tablespoons peanut butter

Fats: 1 tablespoon olive oil, canola oil, or flaxseed oil

Dairy Products: 1 cup milk, 1 cup cottage cheese, 1 ounce or 1 slice of cheese

BREAKFAST

Carbohydrates
● Choose two items.

1 cup Kashi cereal or whole grain cereal

1 piece of whole grain bread (no enriched flour)

1 grapefruit

⅔ cup oatmeal

½ cup grapes

½ cup cantaloupe

½ cup honeydew melon

1 cup low-fat, low-sugar yogurt

1 cup whole grain bran cereal

Protein
● Choose one or two items.

4 egg whites

¼ cup Egg Beaters or other brand egg substitute

2 eggs

1 cup cottage cheese

1 cup 1% milk

3 slices deli meat

2 tablespoons peanut butter

Vegetables
● Choose as many as you like.

1 cup broccoli

1 cup spinach

1 cup green beans

1 cup tomatoes

1 cup cucumbers

1 cup romaine lettuce

1 cup mushrooms

½ cup tomato sauce

Healthy Fats
● Choose one item.

1 tablespoon flaxseed oil

1 to 2 tablespoons olive oil

1 to 2 tablespoons canola oil

¼ cup reduced-fat or low-fat cheese

¼ cup dry-roasted nuts (e.g., almonds)

¼ cup soy nuts

Sample Breakfast

1 cup Kashi cereal and an omelet made with 4 egg whites, veggies, and ¼ cup low-fat cheese.

hand with the winning meal strategies we've already discussed.

- Plan, plan, plan.
- Control the clock.
- Protein + Carbs + Healthy fats.
- Eat to live. Don't live to eat.

Lunch and dinner need not be major productions, especially since you're eating more often. Just take some fish, chicken, or lean red meat; add some vegetables, fruit, or both; and wash it down with two glasses of cold water, or even a glass of red wine. There you have it: a good meal.

As we mentioned earlier, for convenience, you can cook plenty of chicken and fish on Saturdays or Sundays. Buy some prepackaged salads. Put together some vegetables and fruits. The key is to have things ready so you won't be left hungry and scrambling for food, which inevitably results in poor nutritional choices.

The following is a handy guide to assembling your meals and eating properly. It's not an exhaustive list—we provided even more options earlier in this section—but it does give you everything you need to assemble nutritious meals in the least amount of time.

LUNCH OR DINNER

Protein
- Choose one or two items.

4 ounces grilled chicken
1 cup cottage cheese
1 can tuna packed in water
4 ounces skinless turkey
4 ounces lean pork (grilled)
4 ounces grilled lean red meat

Carbohydrates
- Choose one or two.

½ cup brown rice
½ cup whole wheat pasta
½ cup long grain wild rice
1 whole wheat roll
1 slice whole wheat bread

Vegetables
- Choose as many as you like.

1 cup broccoli
1 cup spinach
1 cup green beans
1 cup tomatoes
1 cup cucumbers
1 cup romaine lettuce
1 cup mushrooms
½ cup tomato sauce

Beans and Legumes
- Choose one.

½ cup black beans
½ cup navy beans
½ cup pinto beans
½ cup kidney beans

Low-Glycemic Fruits
- Choose one or two.

1 apple
1 peach
1 plum
1 cup cherries
1 grapefruit
1 pear

Healthy Fats
- Choose one item.

1 to 2 tablespoons olive oil
1 to 2 tablespoons canola oil
¼ cup 2% cheese
¼ cup dry-roasted nuts
(e.g. almonds)
¼ cup soy nuts

Sample Lunch or Dinner

1 cup brown rice and 6 ounces grilled chicken, with a side salad made from 2 cups spinach and 1 cup cucumbers with 2 tablespoons *each* olive oil and vinegar.

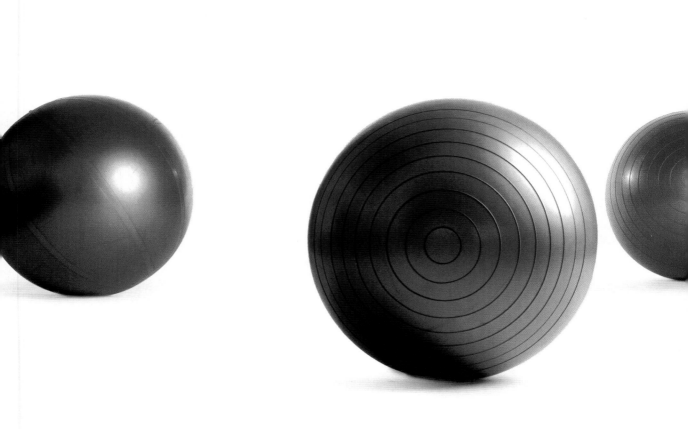

CHAPTER 7

ROAD GAMES

t's always more difficult for a sports team to win on the road than it is at home. After all, the athletes must face the grind of travel, playing in a hostile environment, and not having all of the creature comforts of home.

To compensate, teams stay at the nicest hotels, bring planeloads of equipment, and implement a game plan tailored specifically to the task. The idea is to control the unfamiliar environment as much as possible. Still, in order to succeed, the team must play at a higher level at an opponent's venue. There's little margin for error.

The same is true with nutrition. It's less of a challenge to eat right at home. After all, you've created a home field advantage by stocking the refrigerator and pantry with healthy foods.

You've plotted your meals and snacks around work and weekly routines. You've put your family on notice that you're going to eat healthfully—hopefully getting them to buy into the same program.

Away from home, however, it's much more difficult to eat right. Whether it's a busy day of commitments and errands running around town, a business trip involving air travel and hotel stays, or simply visiting a friend's house for an evening, you will face formidable obstacles to eating right.

So, once again, you should be proactive and plan ahead. At the very least, grab bottled water, fruit, and a bag of nuts before leaving the house. Keep healthy meal-replacement bars in the car, or in your briefcase or backpack. If you're going to be running around all day, pack a healthy salad or a one-serving plastic container with a lean protein source and a vegetable.

In order to stay properly fueled, you must eat roughly every 3 hours, and that's a challenge away from home. We've already discussed how to handle eating at work—think of that MVP drawer and bringing lunch from home—but that's a little easier since work routines are fairly consistent.

There's nothing more counterproductive to a healthy lifestyle than playing goalie when it comes to nutrition. If you're out running errands, chances are you're in a hurry. You lose track of time and the next thing you know, you're driving through a fast-food lane or casing a 7-Eleven or Circle K in search of quick nourishment.

Not only does this wreak havoc on your body but it's also time-consuming, expensive, and frustrating. You don't want to have to pay for the right to eat bad food, and waste time doing it. Plan ahead and you'll save time and money while fueling your body for maximum energy.

Traveling presents another challenge. In re-cent years, airlines have eliminated meal service, which is a good thing because it keeps us from eating highly processed airline food and forces us to be proactive about meal planning. Instead of buying expensive pizza and junk food in the concourse, bring a meal from home. Don't forget the bottled water.

On long car trips, fill a cooler with bottled water, fresh fruit, vegetables, lean protein sources, healthy snack bars, and low-fat, low-sugar yogurt. Graze in the car and stop at rest areas instead of pulling off the highway and frequenting fast-food joints. Again, you'll save time and money in addition to eating right.

For longer trips, whether by car or plane, be sure to take meal-replacement powder to mix into a shake. If you're traveling, instead of lugging around a blender, a far better choice is to use the specifically designed Core Nutrition Shaker Bottle, which gives you a rotator cuff workout in the process! (They're available for less than $10 at many health food stores and at www.coreperformance.com.) Fill a small plastic container with your whey protein, which you can sprinkle onto oatmeal to punch up the protein content, and mix with water and juice for pre-workout shooters. Be sure to pack multivitamins and antioxidants too.

Eating in sit-down restaurants need not be challenging. It's almost always possible to order grilled chicken or fish with vegetables and a salad. Skip the bread and creamy appetizers. If a menu item isn't quite right, you usually have the option of substituting or asking for it to be prepared differently.

No matter what kind of "road game" you encounter, control the environment as much as possible. Plan ahead. Bring all of the equipment you need; it need not weigh you down. Let those other travelers stand in line at the airport for a greasy, $6 piece of pizza. Let others waste their time, money, and health at McDonald's.

We'll talk in the coming chapters about strategies to work out on the road, which people generally find easier than eating right when traveling. But whether it's exercise or nutrition, you can take pride in knowing that you've brought the home field advantage with you.

THE TOUGHEST ROAD GAME

There are certain sports venues that make it almost impossible for a visiting team to win.

BEING A GRACIOUS GUEST

When it comes to nutrition, it's tough to be a gracious guest. Sooner or later, you'll find yourself at a family gathering facing a heaping plate of Aunt Edna's sausage lasagna, buttery garlic bread, and mashed potatoes. Or maybe the boss or a key client has invited you over for spaghetti, spare ribs, or some other fat-laden dish.

I suppose you could fake an upset stomach or declare your allegiance to a special diet, which would be partially true. But either way, you're probably going to offend someone.

Your best bet is to eat a small portion, which will be easier if you're eating six meals a day. Not only that, but you should eat before arriving at the House of Fat. That way you'll feel full and not be inclined to down a bad meal. Another strategy is to bring a dish, even if the host insists they have everything covered. You've saved yourself and contributed to the meal.

It's easier to get by at a casual party. Nobody is going to notice if you don't touch the chips, dips, pizza, burgers, hot dogs, beer, and soda. Like the sit-down dinner situation, it's best to plan ahead and eat before the party or bring dishes to share.

Of course, you could schedule your free day to coincide with the party, which might be the easiest solution. But sometimes there are too many events and not enough free days.

Planning ahead is the best strategy. After all, when it comes to nutrition, sometimes a friendly environment can be hostile territory.

Whether it's the bitter cold of Green Bay's Lambeau Field or Duke University's Cameron Indoor Stadium, with its "Cameron Crazies" that taunt opposing teams, it's tough to win on the road.

The same is true with nutrition. On the road, it's more difficult to eat right. You're generally at the mercy of restaurant menus, and you're usually pressed for time. Ideally, you can still find a healthier restaurant, but there will be times when you end up in the Cameron Indoor Stadium of nutrition: the fast-food joint.

When you enter the opposing venue and see its vast menu of unhealthy yet tempting foods, don't forget your goals: *peak performance and optimal health.* Fast-food restaurants can be a roadblock to your nutrition goals, but with a little planning and some specific requests, you can turn any fast-food-restaurant meal into one that is healthier. Just remember these specific rules, courtesy of our wonderful Amanda Carlson, the nutrition manager and research coordinator at Athletes' Performance:

1. Stay away from the fryer (e.g., fried chicken, french fries, etc). Choose a side salad or baked potato as your side.

2. Go with grilled foods instead.

3. The less legs the better. Grilled chicken or fish is a healthier option than a burger.

4. Remove the skin. If there is skin on your chicken or turkey, take it off.

5. Hold the mayo.

6. Go with water instead of soda or iced tea. Not only is it better for you, it's free.

Think about what you have already eaten throughout the day. Make choices that are low in fat and that contain the right amount of carbohydrates for you. Remember that carbohydrates equal fuel, so if it is earlier in the day or after a workout, you may need more of them. If it is later in the day and less activity is planned, then a reduced amount will do just fine. Consider the following tips to help reduce the amount of processed carbohydrates in your meal:

1. Remove the bun from your burger or chicken sandwich, or remove just the top and eat it open-faced.

2. Order an extra chicken breast for your salad and skip the bun.

3. Leave the croutons off of your salad.

Now, let's take a look at some of the world's toughest venues in which to eat properly and how to make the choices. This list notes the best options offered.

Wendy's

● Wendy's Garden Sensation Salads with a low-fat dressing

- Grilled chicken sandwich and a side salad with a low-fat dressing
- Large chili with a side salad with low-fat dressing
- Small chili and a baked potato with steamed broccoli
- If you must eat a cheeseburger, choose a single with cheese—no mayo.
- Include water with these items. If you must have a soda, choose diet.

Baja Fresh (Mexican Grill)

- Bare Burrito with half the rice
- Baja Ensalada with salsa verde dressing
- Fresh Mahi Mahi Ensalada
- Bean and cheese burrito
- Bean and cheese burrito, add grilled chicken
- Two Chicken Taco Chilitos
- Hold the sour cream; go light on the cheese and guacamole.
- Include water with these items. If you must have soda, choose diet.

Subway

- Six-inch turkey, roast beef, chicken, or ham on whole wheat bread or as a wrap
- Make your sandwich into a salad.

- Skip the cheese or, if you must, go with Swiss cheese.
- Add plenty of vegetables such as tomatoes, pickles, black olives, cucumbers, and green peppers. Go with spinach instead of iceberg lettuce.
- Go light on the mayonnaise.
- Drink water instead of soda.

Any Pizzeria

- Choose a thin-crust vegetable, Hawaiian, or cheese pizza.
- Add grilled chicken, ham, and veggies.
- Do not order breadsticks.
- Order a salad with low-fat dressing on the side instead.

Boston Market

- Honey-glazed ham with steamed vegetable medley and fresh fruit
- Rotisserie turkey (skin removed) with green beans and fresh fruit
- Rotisserie chicken (without the skin) with garlic new potatoes and fresh fruit
- Asian chicken salad with half the dressing and no noodles
- Chicken Carver with no sauce and fresh fruit

- Overall hints: Rotisserie turkey, chicken, or ham (all without the skin); Turkey or Chicken Carver with no sauce; steamed veggies, garlic new potatoes, fruit
- Order water with your meal.

Taco Bell

- Chicken soft tacos
- Bean burrito
- Chicken Burrito Supreme
- Fiesta chicken burrito
- Taco salad with salsa, and without the taco shell and tortilla strips
- Order any burrito or taco "Fresco Style" to decrease calorie and fat content by 25 percent.
- Hold the sour cream; go light on the cheese and guacamole.
- Include water with these items. If you must have a soda, choose diet.

McDonald's

- Chicken McGrill sandwich with BBQ sauce instead of mayo, and a side salad with low-fat vinaigrette dressing
- Grilled chicken Caesar with ½ packet low-fat balsamic vinaigrette instead of Caesar dressing
- Grilled chicken California Cobb salad with ½ packet low-fat balsamic vinaigrette
- Cheeseburger (if you must) with a side salad topped with ½ packet of low-fat balsamic vinaigrette
- Egg McMuffin
- Two scrambled eggs with an English muffin
- Fruit and yogurt parfait

Chipotle Grill or Moe's

- Instead of a burrito, skip the tortilla and order a Burrito Bol.
- Decline the sour cream.
- Go with light cheese and guacamole.
- Go to www.ChipotleFan.com to build your virtual burrito and calculate its nutrient value.

Sit-Down Restaurants

- Choose grilled chicken or fish.
- If choosing a steak, trim the fat and choose cuts with less marbling.
- Start with a salad with low-fat dressing.
- Choose steamed vegetables as sides.
- Eat rolls and potato dishes in moderation.

An overall lifestyle of healthy choices improves health and performance. Healthy eating habits overpower one not-so-great choice.

Chapter 7 Summary: Eating on the road presents a number of challenges. The key, once again, is proper planning. Stock your car, desk, briefcase, backpack, or diaper bag with healthy options so you won't have to turn to junk food when things get hectic. You need not eat poorly at sit-down restaurants. Go with grilled chicken or fish and steamed vegetables. If you must eat at a fast-food restaurant, make the best possible choice.

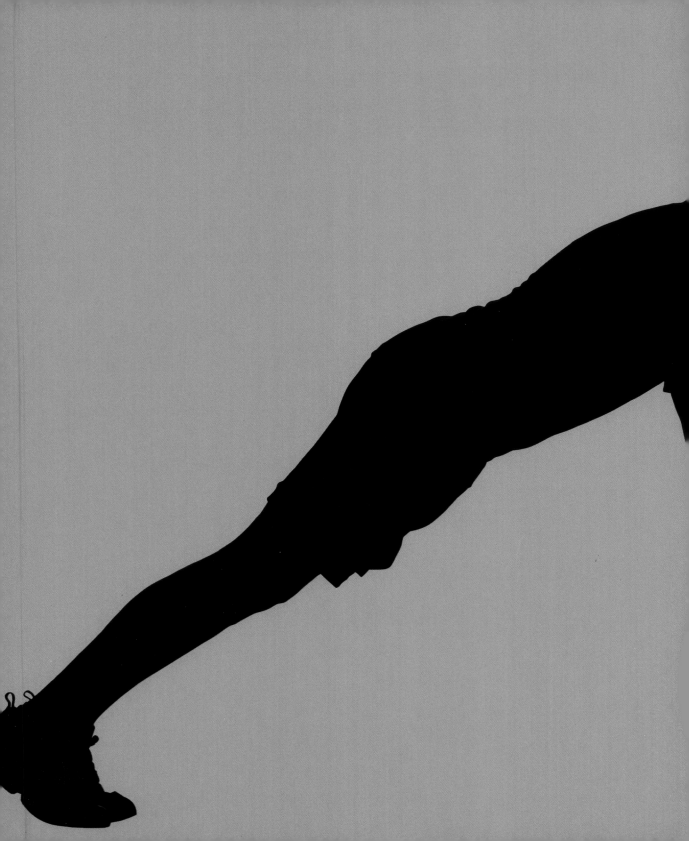

CORE
MOVEMENT

MINDSET

NUTRITION

MOVEMENT

RECOVERY

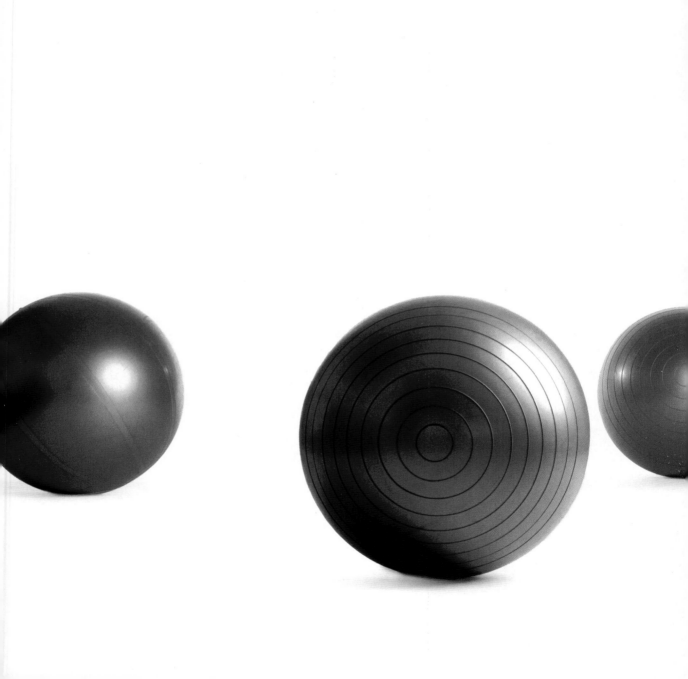

BUILDING YOUR INNER CORE

When you people-watch at the mall or airport, it's easy to tell who's in shape and who's not. We make the same judgments when we look at ourselves in the mirror. If you are committed and resilient with the Core program, your body will undergo a physical transformation. But I need you to think not just in terms of the way you look but also in terms of the way you *move.*

When I watch people, the first thing I notice is their movement patterns. I might see them walking with one or both of their feet rotating outward, which prevents them from rolling over on their toes or using their ankle joints. That leads to tight ankles, hips, and lower-back pain.

Other times, I notice a person's hip instability. With every step they take, they put undue stress upon and cause excess wear of the knees, feet, groin, and, by extension, the spine.

In the short term, this might not seem like anything other than soreness after a long day of walking. Down the road, however, one of those areas will become a major problem.

These people, some of whom are in decent shape, suffer from "biomechanical dysfunction." From a height/weight standpoint, they might look like they're in above-average condition, but they still have biomechanical dysfunction because they no longer can perform the necessary movements to thrive and sustain a high quality of life. Maybe they don't realize it now, but they will when something breaks down. It's like driving your car when the wheels aren't aligned.

At our training centers we conduct an analysis of each athlete's movement-pattern efficiency. The idea is to make sure they meet and exceed the excruciating demands of their sports. We also take a look at the athletes' software—in other words, *their brains*. The Game of Life installs viruses into our software through injury and illness, lack of activity, and improper training. We need to improve the way our software boots up so that our bodies operate efficiently to create functional, fluid movement that protects and propels us.

We do this by trying to determine which, if any, muscles are "overfiring," creating tightness and tension, and by seeing whether any muscles have been turned off all together. This causes other muscles to overcompensate, leading to muscle fatigue and strain.

When we get these movement patterns working properly, we find a body that is perfectly balanced to efficiently store and release energy with every step. These graceful patterns allow muscles to complement one another, smoothly transferring energy back and forth; they feed off one another in perfect harmony. This program will help you achieve the same feeling.

Most exercise programs provide the standard workouts that you equate with traditional fitness. Many people see exercise solely in the one-dimensional, old-school mode. Authors and followers of such programs might belittle you for your willingness to try something new, going beyond the stale, inefficient regimens at the gym. But by using the Core program, you will be able to reach your fitness goals better than the majority of people exercising at clubs—and often better than their trainers, who believe people should follow the same program they use every day.

The movements you'll learn through the Core program might seem unusual, but they're effective. They are derivatives of the guiding principles we use at Athletes' Performance. We can't take credit for these powerful movements because they are merely variations of childhood movement; they just need dusting off.

As a baby, you started to learn these movement patterns, first by rolling over. Gradually, you began to crawl, stand, squat, walk, and run. You progressed during the preteen and teenage years, refining these movement patterns to higher levels. And then what happened? You stopped progressing, falling into a less active lifestyle of school, work, and screen time. That is where you left off, and that's where we will begin.

At first, this program might seem remedial as we return to the basics of movement, but be patient. Don't get frustrated as you learn these new exercises. Give yourself some time. Like a

Have you written down a consistent, weekly plan that is realistic and achievable given the time constraints in your life?

Do you define the success of your exercise program primarily by the changes you see in the mirror?

Do you know how your program improves your body function so that you can thrive given the demands of the Game of Life?

Does your program create pain as much as, if not more than, it reduces pain?

Does travel, the demands of your job or family, or another external factor throw you off of your program?

baby, we will learn and steadily progress throughout your lifespan.

We have broken up these exercises into four simple categories:

● Movement Preparation (or "Movement Prep")

● Prehabilitation (or "Prehab")

● Strength and Performance Circuits

● Cardio

These four categories or "players" are important individually and even more so as a comprehensive regimen. They might have you off-balance at first, but the athlete inside of you will adjust to meet the challenge.

In part 4, we will add a fifth element called Regeneration. Think of Regeneration as a closer in baseball—the guy who gets those final outs and seals the deal. This element will allow you to catch your breath, and it will encourage all the benefits of the four preceding elements to take effect. That way, when I call you back into the game tomorrow, you will

be able to improve on your last performance.

First, I want you to toss aside everything you know about exercise. The problem with most workout routines is that they're based on bodybuilding. You work your biceps and triceps on one day, your legs the next. But unless your goals are to take up residence in a gym and win bodybuilding championships, you're wasting time and not improving overall health. Before you get started, take the time to answer questions in the Core Movement Assessment above.

In this chapter, you will learn to adopt a realistic exercise plan that you'll be able to stick to regardless of the demands of work, family, and travel. You'll see why it does not make sense to define fitness by how you look in the mirror but rather by your body's function and how resistant it is to injury and long-term deterioration.

Like the rest of the program, we want to focus on the centered self and build from the inside out. Not only that, but we're now thinking of ourselves as athletes, and athletes do not train with the intent of improving their looks.

They train in order to master the movements that their sports require. We need to train the same way to compete in the Game of Life.

You might think that your daily movements do not require much athleticism—and oh, how wrong you are. What about lifting children or groceries? What about reacting quickly and maintaining balance when you slip on a wet floor? How about climbing stairs, rushing to grab a taxi or subway, or working in the yard?

All of these things require athletic, *functional* movement. If you're going to invest the time to work out, why not do it with more than aesthetics in mind? By following the Core Workout and Nutrition program, you'll train your body, and as an added bonus, you'll get in phenomenal shape—in far less time than bodybuilders spend in the gym.

Bodybuilding-based workouts view the physique as a series of parts, and most people tend to think of movement as starting from the limbs. If we reach out to grab something or step forward, we think of those motions as originating with the end result—we've reached out, therefore, we've used our arms.

But movement starts from the very center of the body, the core area of the torso. That's why we refer to the torso as the *pillar*—it's the structural center of movement and life. The way we maintain that pillar—its alignment and function—directly correlates to the health of our organs and the rest of our bodies. Everything is interrelated.

PILLAR STRENGTH

Pillar strength is the foundation of all movement. It consists of hip, core, and shoulder stability. (If you're having a hard time getting your head around this concept, it might help to picture your body as a mannequin with no limbs.) Those three areas give us a center axis from which to move. If you think of the body as a wheel, the pillar is the hub, and the limbs are spokes.

We want to have the hub perfectly aligned so we can draw energy from it and effectively transfer energy throughout the body. It's impossible to move the limbs efficiently and forcefully if they're not attached to something solid and stable.

There's a reason why parents are forever telling kids to sit up straight. Without pillar strength, without what I call "perfect posture," you will significantly increase the potential for injury in a chain that starts with your lower back, descends all the way to the knees and ankles, and rises up to your neck, shoulders, and elbows.

The reason we train body *movements* instead of parts is because everything about the body's engineering is connected. What happens to the big toe affects the knees, the hips, and ultimately the shoulders. The muscular system is both complex and simple, a series of muscular and fascial bands that work seamlessly to produce efficient movement. Many workout programs do more damage than good by producing muscle imbalances and inefficient movement patterns that sabotage this highly coordinated operating system that we're born with.

Remember the way that movement evolves in infants. They move on their backs until one day this action allows them to roll over, initiating the hip crossover movement. Soon they progress to crawling, standing, and, finally, walking. With each step, they realize how to stabilize their bodies.

Aging reverses that process. Many people lose the ability to squat and maintain their balance, creating poor posture. Eventually, they lose the ability to stand, surrendering the core fundamental movement patterns they developed as toddlers. But instead of conceding that devolution as an unavoidable part of aging, why not look at getting older as a process of taking these movements to new levels? In this program, you're going to take your body to the highest levels of performance and movement capabilities by challenging yourself to increase flexibility and stability. We'll help you do this by adding resistance or increasing the balance demands. This will put you farther and farther away from the regression of aging.

Look, I'm not here to bash bodybuilding and tell you not to lift weights. This program includes resistance training because of its undeniable benefits. The Movement Prep and Prehab routines you'll learn are not a cutesy program to ram the concept of functional exercise down your throat. It's more about repro-gramming the body to function properly—as nature intended—and to continually become stronger. It's possible to become physically stronger every day of our lives.

Instead of looking at movement as coming out of the arms and legs, remember this perfect posture. If you can master the following three elements of pillar strength—shoulder stability, core stability, and hip stability—both while working out and in everyday movement, you will go a long way toward a healthier life.

SHOULDER STABILITY

Anyone who participates in a sport involving hitting or throwing understands the importance of the rotator cuff. It's even more important in everyday life.

We tend to think of the hands and arms as carrying the workload for the upper body, but it's really the shoulder, or at least it should be. After all, we think of someone *shouldering* a burden.

The shoulder "girdle" consists of the humerus, scapula, and clavicle. It's engineered for a remarkable range of three-dimensional movement. From the shoulder, it's possible to rotate, press, and pull. We can raise our arms to the side or across the body. We can rotate shoulders by holding the elbows in and by moving the hands up and in—or in a 90-degree angle to the torso.

Our natural instinct is to drop the shoulders

THE AMISH WORKOUT?

You probably wouldn't think of the Amish as a very athletic people. But because they work mostly as farmers and shun technology, spending no time in front of computers and televisions, they actually are among the fittest.

A recent study of physical activity and body composition in an Old Order Amish community by the American College of Sports Medicine (ACSM) suggests that a large decline in work-related physical activity in North America is a major contributing factor to the obesity epidemic.

Ninety-eight Amish adults in a southern Ontario farming community wore pedometers and logged their physical activities for 7 days. The conservative Amish use 19th-century farming techniques that require physical labor. Not surprisingly, the study indicated that a high level of physical activity is integrated into the daily lives of the Amish.

Amish men reported an average of 10 hours of vigorous work per week and took an average of 18,425 steps a day. Amish women, most of whom work as homemakers, still logged an average of 14,196 daily steps. On average, the Amish participated in roughly *six times* the amount of weekly physical activity performed by nearly 2,000 participants in a recent survey in 12 modernized nations.

"The Amish were able to show us just how far we've fallen in the last 150 years or so in terms of the amount of physical activity we typically perform," says David R. Bassett, professor at the University of Tennessee who served as lead researcher for the study. "Their lifestyle indicates that physical activity played a critical role in keeping our ancestors fit and healthy."

The ACSM study found that only 4 percent of the Amish surveyed were obese and only 26 percent were overweight. Compare that with the United States, where 31 percent of adults are obese and 64.5 percent are overweight.

Because of their high activity levels, the Amish stay fit despite a high-fat, high-sugar diet of meat, potatoes, gravy, eggs, vegetables, bread, pies, and cakes.

If you log 10 laborious hours a week pushing a plow or lifting heavy beams, feel free to enjoy the "Amish Diet." But wouldn't it be easier to accomplish the same level of fitness by tweaking your diet and spending one-third of the time working out?

---

forward, especially after long periods of sitting. But you want to do the opposite, bringing the shoulders back and down, which will give you proper posture.

Remember *The Karate Kid*? Mr. Miyagi, the wise martial arts instructor, made his young student Daniel LaRusso paint his fence and wax his cars. For days this went on and Daniel wondered if he was ever going to learn karate. When he confronted Miyagi, the old man asked him to demonstrate the various motions of painting and waxing and then attacked Daniel from all angles. Using the same motions, Daniel easily defended himself and quickly realized that he had not just been painting and waxing but stabilizing and strengthening his shoulder muscles and mastering these vital, functional movements.

If you're involved in martial arts, this program will help by stabilizing your shoulders—and I won't make you wax cars and paint houses. Even if you have no desire to become the next Bruce Lee or Chuck Norris, you must strengthen this area to perform everyday activities from cleaning to passing objects to filing to, yes, waxing and painting.

Most of us don't realize how hunched over we are from sitting at computers and traveling in cars and airplanes. People tend to think that this affects only the elderly, but that's not the case. The next time you're people-watching at a mall or airport, pay attention to the position of their thumbs. If they're rotated in, pointing toward the body, that means their heads and shoulders have moved forward.

Unless those people do something, I guarantee that they will soon have rotator cuff and back problems, which will limit their ability to participate in the daily activities of life.

As people age, they tend to flex forward, as if the chest is caving in. We want to do the opposite, almost as if there's a fishhook inserted under the sternum, pulling us up. This will allow the shoulders to fall into place and help give perfect posture.

We're not trying to be military cadets, standing at attention. Instead, think of this as standing or sitting tall in a comfortable position, always elevating the sternum.

The exercises in this program will require you to bring the shoulders back and down, but you'll want to make it a daily habit. To make lasting change, we want to lengthen the chest and strengthen the muscles of the upper back. Think of pulling your shoulders toward your back pockets. This posture is the exact opposite of the shoulder shrug, the same motion that you make when you say, "I don't know." That's what a sitting lifestyle does to you. If you create a habit of bringing your shoulders down, you'll be amazed at the results. People will find you more confident and think you've lost weight because you're no longer slouched over. They might even think you've grown. There have been instances of adults following this program and gaining up to an inch of height from standing tall and bringing their shoulders back, as well as improving hip and core stability.

CORE STABILITY

The middle third of our pillar is the "core," which consists of the muscles of the abdominals, torso, and lower back. It's the vital link between shoulder and hip stability, and it includes such muscle groups as the rectus abdominis, transversus abdominis, internal and external obliques, lats, the erector spinae, and many small stabilizer muscles between the vertebrae of the spine.

These are the tiny muscles that often get shut off because of a back injury and never become reactivated, causing long-term back problems. These small stabilizer muscles cannot function alone; they must be helped by training the muscles of the core to become strong and stable with the right types of recruitment patterns that will enable them to work in tandem with the shoulders and hips.

Core training is *not* just about the abs—abs are less than a third of the equation. Countless books and magazine articles promise great abs, and though many of them have terrific exercises that we believe in, they're of little use unless done in conjunction with exercises aimed at integrating your shoulders and hips.

Instead of just focusing on the abs, we want to create the framework for all movement. The aim isn't just a well-sculpted midsection; it's a high-performance core.

In order to maximize the benefit of the exercises in this book, it's important to keep your tummy tight, not just while exercising but all day. Think of your tummy flat against the hip bones. Keep your tummy tight, as if pulling your belly button off the belt buckle. This isn't the same as sucking in your gut and holding your breath. Keep the abdominals in, but still breathe.

The abdominal and lower-back muscles work as a team. The point guard is the transverse abdominis, which is the first muscle that's recruited each time you move. If you can keep that "TA" activated and your tummy tight, you'll be well on your way to optimum movement and preventing long-term deterioration.

HIP STABILITY

All of those muscles that attach to your ribs and spine are extremely important for shoulder and core stability. But what good would this be without a strong foundation?

In all the people I evaluate, including the best athletes in the world, the number one focus is hip function and stability—in other words, how they use their pelvis. If people better understood how to use the pelvis and hips, we could eradicate lower-back pain, knee pain, foot ailments, and a host of other aches that make us miserable.

We tend to think that if our ankles, knees, or feet hurt, there must be something wrong with those areas. But if we again look at the body as a wheel, the pillar, and more specifically, the pelvis, is the hub of that wheel. The pelvis is in charge of controlling the spokes. You might have the greatest spokes (legs and thighs), but if something goes wrong with the hub, the spokes cannot function.

Many injuries are caused by hip tightness and a lack of hip stability. As a result, the body does not recruit the necessary muscles from the pelvic region, and it puts more stress on other areas, which overcompensate and get injured.

We want to go to the source of the problem and prevent injuries from happening. On either

"My pain just seemed to dissipate."

NAME: JAIME MERRIFIELD

AGE: 45

HOMETOWN: MESA, ARIZONA

Jaime Merrifield was an avid triathlete until she was diagnosed several years ago with chronic fatigue syndrome, chronic mononucleosis, and fibromyalgia, a musculoskeletal pain and fatigue disorder characterized by pain in the muscles, ligaments, and tendons.

She's not sure exactly what brought on the health problems, but she has a few ideas. At age 11, she dove off her father's shoulders and hit her head on the bottom of a swimming pool. As a young adult, doctors told her she had the spine of a football player, so compressed were her vertebrae. She chalked that up to a bicycle accident at age 23 and the stress from long hours spent standing as a teacher.

"I would seem healthy and fit and then I'd crash for a month and sleep," she says. "People thought I was lazy, but it turned out I have these chronic conditions."

The ailments were devastating for an active working mom in her midforties who has a busy schedule as a veterinarian. She had tried other exercise programs only to give up when the pain became too much. With the Core program, she found the pain manageable. In fact, some of her chronic pain began to dissipate.

"What I like about the program is the combination of light weights and stretching," she says. "The key is the order in which you do them. I've done variations of a lot of it independently, using a physioball and doing Pilates, but this has proven to be the best mix. It's helped so much both mentally and physically."

Merrifield found the Movement Prep routine especially beneficial.

"You get that endorphin release, and my pain just seemed to dissipate. I stopped getting so many migraines."

As a veterinarian and a pain sufferer, Jaime has studied what causes pain and the links to depression. It's no surprise to find that anyone suffering from chronic pain might feel depressed, but Jaime believes that research in the coming years will show a neurological link between the two.

"People will tell you they suffered depression after a major injury, and that's no coincidence," she says. "It's a vicious cycle. I've found there's something in the way the exercises of the Core program are arranged that has proven, at least for me, to really inhibit those pain triggers."

As a triathlete, Jaime always valued an active lifestyle, and she suffered when that was taken away from her. Now, she views training as a necessity just to get through her days.

"If I miss a day or two, I feel like I don't want to get out of bed," she says. "If this program can have this kind of impact on someone like me, I can only imagine the positive effects it could have on others."

side of the pelvis is a hip "capsule," where the femur attaches to the pelvis. This along with more than 40 muscles in and around this hip capsule creates the "hip cuff." This should allow you to rotate your knees in or all the way out, as well as lifting your leg up or back and in every combination. You should be able to lift a leg up and across your body, as if posing for the Heisman Trophy.

Most people get into trouble squatting by using their quadriceps rather than the muscles of the hips to initiate movement. As a result, the knees slide forward, the glutes (your butt) don't get involved, and there's undue pressure on the knees and back. Our goal is to become more glute-dominant. Watch kids and see how well they squat and stand up. Many of us have lost this movement from sitting too much and being inactive.

Thankfully, we can get it back. Let's practice for a moment. From a standing position, place your feet farther than hip width apart. Lean forward, arms straight ahead. Elevate your chest by feeling tall and pulling your shoulders toward the back pockets and keep your tummy tight. Now, try and sit with the hips; instead of flopping down, as you might if there was a chair underneath, sit firmly by using your hips. Try to create an arch in your lower back, shifting the weight to the middle part of your foot, even a little toward the heel. Feel the glutes and the other muscles of your hip capsule stretch as you lower your body. Squeeze your glutes to stand back up.

Now try to push your pelvis forward while standing and *then* squat. It doesn't work because you drive the knees over the toes. No wonder so many people suffer from knee injuries.

We want to initiate all movement from the hips, while maintaining perfect posture. If you're going up steps, squatting to pick something up, or simply standing up, squeeze your glutes until your legs are extended. Walk with your toes pointed forward, your chest over your knee, and push through your hips until your leg is extended. That might mean you have to skip every other step, but that's okay. This way, the pressure is on your hips—where nature intended—not the knees.

The reason we see so many running-related injuries is because people don't have the necessary hip stability. Runners have to be able to effectively balance on a single leg and move from the hips. If the hips don't stabilize, the force created by the pounding of running is stored in the body. That energy is absorbed and stored in the muscles, tendons, and joints, leading to overuse injuries.

But if you're stable in the hips, core, and shoulders, the energy transfers through the feet, legs, core, and through the opposite arm, leading to maximum performance. So, by creating a mobile and stabile hip joint, you will store and release energy efficiently, creating optimum movement.

A properly functioning pair of hip capsules is the most powerful thing you have in your body, but it's the most destructive if it's locked down. If your hip capsule is locked down, lacking stability and mobility, it's as if a bone is welded to the pelvis—it's like having a cast on your hip. To get anything to move, you need to have excessive motion in your back and knees. But the better job you do of creating stability, mobility, and strength around the hip, the less potential there is for injury and the far better chance you'll have of performing well in any activity you do.

But the benefit of initiating movement with your hips doesn't stop there. You know the easiest way to get buns of steel? Use them constantly. Don't do just one isolated workout. People who have flat, shapeless butts do not use their hips and glutes properly in everyday movement; they just have a couple of saggy bags back there. Look for every opportunity to lengthen and strengthen those glutes, whether it's squatting, going up stairs, getting out of a chair, or simply walking. It's the foundation for all movement.

Think of life as one big glute workout and you'll see amazing results. Every time you walk, move and bend, fire (squeeze) those glutes. Don't take them for granted.

One way to keep track of how active you're becoming in day-to-day life is simply to use a pe-dometer. These easy-to-use devices, available for $10 or less, keep track of how many steps you take. At the end of the day, you can see how much you moved—or did not move—and that's terrific motivation to turn your daily routines into more of a workout. Adidas, one of my company's sponsors, even has a new "MOVE" shoe with a pedometer built into the heel that calculates your steps throughout the day. The MOVE, due out in February 2006, features a digital readout with seven digits to count up to 9,999,999 steps. If you make it to that point, you definitely will have made your life a daily workout—to say nothing of needing a new pair of shoes!

Remember, you're a competitive athlete in the Game of Life, and that's not just when you're working out. Throughout the day, fire those glutes, keep that tummy tight, and elevate the chest. Soon you'll be gliding through life like the successful person you are.

Chapter 8 Summary: Effective workouts train the body for athletic, functional movement. It's about training *movements,* not body parts. Pillar strength, the foundation of movement, consists of shoulder, core, and hip stability.

Try to work these areas beyond your workout routine. Make it a daily habit to bring your shoulders back and down as if you're putting them in your back pockets. Keep your tummy tight, and fire those glutes.

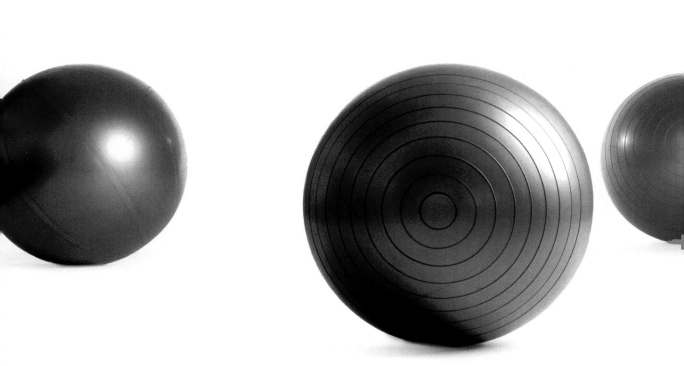

CHAPTER 9

THE CORE WORKOUT: AN INTRODUCTION

Everything in a professional athlete's life is accelerated. A single play, game, season, or career can be a microcosm of the Game of Life. It's about teamwork and competition. There are challenges and adjustments and, ultimately, wins and losses.

An athlete's career is especially accelerated—most ballplayers attempt to stretch their careers out to the age of 35 or 40, though most end long before that. Athletes constantly try to improve their skills and have a small window of opportunity to take advantage of them. Yet no matter how well they've done this, they've accelerated the aging process. Their bodies have been driven so hard and crashed so many times, it's as if they've been artificially aged.

This is no different from our own lives. For most of us, competitive athletics ends in Little League, high school, or college. Even those who make it into the pros have a career lifespan of just 3½ years on average. Some find a way to last 10 to 15 years and walk away from the game still ready to enjoy the fruits of all their hard work.

Your working career will last 40 years, perhaps longer. Thankfully, you need not endure the punishment of a football player, the grind of marathon training, or the repetitive stress a pitcher's shoulder undergoes. Yet your deterioration is no different, just more gradual and subtle. By sitting at computers all day and remaining inactive, you lose mobility. Joints begin to lock down, and over time, you develop excruciating hip and back problems.

By not taking action now, you're not only ensuring this decline, you're expediting the process—to the point that, at all of 45 years old, you may have inflicted as much damage on your body as someone who's spent a decade playing in the NFL.

I have friends between the ages of 35 and 55 who say that it hurts to get in and out of a car. They avoid squatting because it hurts their knees and back. It saddens me because they've lost part of what makes them who they are. Instead of being vibrant, happy, pain-free people, they've aged long before their time.

Research into aging suggests that while we might not be able to live decades longer by taking care of our bodies, we can dramatically improve the quality of our remaining years. That's a key part of the Core philosophy. It's not just about the length of time, it's about the *quality* of our time. This program arrests the natural decline of aging, helping you master the fundamental skills you've probably forgotten. We're going to turn on those transmitters that have been shut off from spending too much time at your desk and off your feet.

It all starts with the notion of activating your core, as discussed in the last chapter. You want to keep your shoulders pulled back and down and your tummy tight. You also want to initiate movement from your hips and glutes.

If you suffer from back or joint pain, haven't exercised in years, and possess a lack of energy and muscle tightness, you're going to get out of the rut by using some of the same simple principles we use with world-class athletes, but don't be intimidated by that. Many of the athletes we see have the same problems you do. It's just that the stresses of their sports have expedited the process.

I want you to look at *Core Performance Essentials* as the on-ramp to the performance superhighway. The farther down we go on that highway, the farther away we are from aging and deconditioning. It's never too early to jump on the highway. I hope that kids follow this program, too, since they're more susceptible to premature aging than previous generations because of a lack of activity, more screen time, and exposure to processed and fast foods. If kids can master this program, they will rank among the top 10 percent of youth in terms of fitness. Should they want to play sports, this will put them far ahead of the game, and ready for the highest levels of competition. Even if they don't want to play sports, they'll be on the highway toward a long and healthy life. Studies suggest that obese kids become obese adults. The Core program gives us a way to prevent that. There's always been a school of thought that kids should avoid resistance training, since their bones are still growing. But look at how young kids move: They jump off a playground slide or climb monkey bars. There are more forces on joints and musculature in those movements than we could ever create with resistance training. This workout is great for kids, but like anything else, there must be a level of mastery and progression. We're not going to hand a kid—or an adult—a huge weight without teaching him how to perform the movement properly using only his body weight.

Most people remain motivated to work out through the teenage and early adult years, if only because they have more time and are looking to impress potential mates. Once you factor a full-time job into the equation, it becomes more difficult, but you can still make the time.

Some people slack off from fitness once they've found a mate or started a family, but that should be only the *beginning* of a lifelong commitment to health. Now you have responsibility for someone other than yourself. Between a spouse, home ownership, and perhaps children, you have even more reasons to want to ensure that you'll be around for a long time.

As the pace of life increases exponentially because of the demands of having a family—including taking care of kids and, perhaps, elderly parents—life becomes more hectic. Time becomes more precious, and you need this workout solution to maintain the quality of your life.

Time is the only limiting factor. It's the downfall of many fitness programs because there's no progression. People do the same exercises until their bodies are so used to the program that there's no longer a benefit. In some cases, they've made matters worse by creating muscle imbalances. With *Core Performance Essentials,* the progression is unlimited. You're not going to be that person in the gym doing the same routine with the same weight at the same time year after year. The more you progress, the more movements you're able to integrate. Results increase, and in less time.

It's like the Japanese concept of *Kaizen,* which we translate in this country as "continuous improvement." In America, we tend to look for quick fixes and dramatic turnarounds, whether in business or fitness. There's nothing wrong with that mentality, but it often does not come with a foundation for long-term success.

Kaizen strives for steady, uninterrupted, incremental change. It's originally a Buddhist term meaning "Renew the heart and make it good," and that's a literal encapsulation of exactly what we're doing. We're renewing the heart and the rest of the body by increasing its capacity, making it as good and productive as it can be.

Each day, we'll take tiny steps by increasing the amount of weight, the complexity of the movement, or the number of repetitions. We can increase the challenge of balancing by going from two legs to one or by incorporating a physioball. By increasing the "work density," we continually progress by getting more quality work done in less time.

Work density is a key component of this program. In many bodybuilding-based exercise regimens, your work density is limited. You perform 1 set and then rest for at least that long, perhaps while spotting someone, before doing another. As a result, you learn to pace yourself. That's not the case with the Core Workout, because you're constantly moving. And as you become more proficient with the movements, you will do more in less time, thus enabling you either to add more exercises, circuits, reps, or simply perform advanced versions of the ones you're already doing. Either way, you're constantly progressing with the same investment of time.

You can customize the schedule to fit your needs. If you want to work out at home with no equipment, fine. If you have limited access to equipment on the road, we'll show you what to do. Maybe you'd like to invest in a home gym to save time commuting to a gym. Instead of paying around $50 a month in gym fees, take that money and assemble your own home Core Gym at www.coreperformance.com.

We've tested the equipment on the Web site at Athletes' Performance, and we have added significant value by giving you higher-quality equipment, which includes educational DVDs with each product to show you how to get the most out of it, and how you may integrate this into the Core program. That allows you to keep mixing things up and progressing using the same effective system.

These versatile, inexpensive pieces of equipment, such as mini bands, elastic tubing home gyms, adjustable dumbbells, slideboard tops, physioballs, medicine balls, and foam rolls, don't take up a large amount of space. We've also engineered this system to adapt and grow with your needs. Recognizing that there will be times when you're limited by a lack of equipment, we've provided options. Here, then, are the four units of the Core Workout.

MOVEMENT PREPARATION

Movement Preparation is an active series of warmup exercises that will efficiently increase your core temperature, lengthen, strengthen, stabilize, and balance your muscles, and, as the name suggests, prepare the body for movement.

Perhaps you're accustomed to performing static, stretch-and-hold exercises that seem like a precursor to actually working out. That's not the case with Movement Prep. As with everything else in the Core Workout, you're making the most of your time. You're warming up and preparing for movement, but this is part of the actual workout. In fact, if you ever get to the end of the day and realize that you have not worked out, do the Movement Prep routine. If you're that pressed for time, you can at least make this 5-minute investment in your long-term health.

With Movement Prep, you're going to both lengthen and strengthen your muscles in the same movement. Movement Prep will re-estab-

CORE SUCCESS STORY
"Haven't felt this good since I was 9!"

NAME: MARSHALL VINER

AGE: 42

HOMETOWN: WHISTLER, BRITISH COLUMBIA

Marshall Viner figured his days as an active athlete were over. He spent his teenage years playing hockey and working in the physically taxing business of commercial fishing, straining his back to lift nets and hoist fish. At 18, he endured a horrific toboggan accident, landing on his spine.

Doctors told him he never would play sports again and that he would endure back trouble for the rest of his life. Eventually, he was diagnosed with juvenile discogenic disease, a degenerative spinal condition that causes excruciating back pain.

Through the years, Viner has endured surgeries, visited chiropractors, and undergone agonizing physical therapy. All helped, to some degree. But he still could not run without feeling pain in his hips and back.

His job as a real estate agent involves lunches with clients and late dinners. Soon, he had packed 190 pounds onto his 5-foot-5 frame, which only exacerbated his back problems.

Then, Viner tried the Core program and found that he could run without pain. Soon he was running 30 to 40 miles a week on a treadmill. He lost 20 pounds.

"It feels so good to be this mobile," Viner says. "My back hasn't felt this good since I was 9!"

Viner finds it most effective to do some Core training after swimming or treadmill work. "It's given me phenomenal results," he says. "I wish I had known about this program 20 years ago. A lot of people suffer from back pain and figure there's nothing they can do about it. That's not the case. You've got to find a way to keep moving. This program has showed me how."

lish the mobility, coordination, and joint stability you enjoyed in your younger years and it's going to improve strength, balance, and coordination—in other words, it will heighten your body's ability to process information.

This is not about developing rippling abdominal muscles to support your lower back—that's just one piece of the puzzle. Instead, you're going to perform the fundamental movements necessary to sustain and enjoy life, re-

establishing the chains that were broken as you became less active.

You want to improve the long-term mobility and flexibility of muscles. Rather than have them stretch and go back to where they were—as is the case with traditional stretch-and-hold routines—you want your body to remember these new ranges of motion.

This is done through a process of lengthening the muscle (known as active elongation), which is more effective than a traditional stretch. Here's the crucial difference: After you stretch the muscle to this new range of motion, you stabilize, then contract through the new range of motion. In other words, you don't just stretch your muscles and let them snap back into place, like a rubber band. Instead, you show your muscles how to use the motion.

I don't care how out of shape or tight you are. No matter how much your knees or back hurt, you can do the exercises listed in Level 1. There are no excuses. So many people refuse to work out because they have such ailments, and that only leads to more discomfort. By not working out, you will hurt more, and your quality of life will deteriorate. If you just follow this Movement Prep routine, however, you will eliminate the symptoms and thus your excuses for not exercising. All it takes is a desire to move better and experience less pain.

Once you've mastered Movement Prep, you will know the Core movements you need to protect your body from the long-term deterioration of aging.

PREHAB

That brings us to the concept of what I call Prehab. You're no doubt familiar with rehabilitation, or "rehab," which often is needed to recover from injuries brought about from a lack of movement or exercise.

With the Prehab routine, you're going to protect your body from backsliding into the pain, inactivity, and dysfunction that lead to the downward spiral. Prehab is a valuable insurance policy. If you do nothing else but Movement Prep and Prehab, you will maintain the physical abilities you need to lead an engaged, full, active life. (You should, however, add the Strength and Cardio units to the mix to maximize energy and long-term health.)

Wherever life takes you, Prehab is something you can do in a few minutes each day to maintain your body. This routine (see page 141) protects you from shoulder pain, lower-back trouble, hip pain, and knee and foot ailments. It will give you the necessary balance, coordination, strength, and endurance to function in everyday life.

Prehab, along with Movement Prep, will give you the basic requirements for all human movement, the absolute minimum to sustain quality of life. And yet, 90 percent of Americans cannot perform these basic movements. Master Prehab and you'll be among the top.

Regardless of how crazy life gets, make time to do your Prehab exercises just three times a week. As long as you can perform Movement Prep and Prehab, you will be well-prepared to face middle age and your senior years. You will be less likely to endure crippling back pain and hip ailments, which may cause both premature aging and entry into an assisted-living facility down the road.

That's the problem with most workout routines. They get you in shape for short-term goals, but there's no long-term vision. If you're only motivated by a college reunion, a wedding, or the upcoming swimsuit season, you'll be far less likely to make a lasting commitment. Let those events be motivational—for what you want to look and feel like for the rest of your life.

Even pro athletes are guilty of this short-sightedness. Their careers end and they stop all activity. It's amazing how often you see a former baseball player hobble onto the field to be honored before a game. Inevitably, he's packed on 30 pounds and struggles just to trot out to wave to the crowd.

But at least that guy probably stayed active into his late thirties. Most people quit long before that, retiring from the Game of Life well before their prime. If only they had invested some time in Prehab.

Remember that Prehab is not a short-term solution. You will experience immediate results, to be sure, but there needs to be a long-term commitment. Nothing less than your long-term health and quality of life is at stake.

This is true of the entire Core program: It's a progression, and if you want great results, you have to stick with it. First, we stop the bad habits of poor eating and inactivity, thus decreasing your pain. That's where the Core Nutrition chapter and Movement Prep came in. Now we're going to help you become active, thus preventing future pain. And that's the beauty of Prehab: You will be investing in your long-term health and productivity, which leads to a strong performance in the Game of Life.

STRENGTH

Once we've mastered the Movement Prep and Prehab routines, we're going to add some strength training. Isn't it interesting that people always refer to *weight* training, not strength training? After all, you're training to become stronger.

Too many people lift the same weights, week after week, and year after year. Their bodies adapt and stop getting stronger. These people probably follow bodybuilding-based programs that make no effort to work the core or to train for functional movement.

We, however, will focus on multijoint movements that improve coordination and recruit lots of muscles, a process that expends more energy and gives more return on our investment of time. It will burn calories and improve balance, stability, flexibility, strength, and the cardiovascular system all at once.

This is where you become more and more efficient. As you master these movements, you'll find that they take less time. By training in a circuit, alternating movements that emphasize different regions of the body, you will be in constant motion.

If you work out in a gym, you'll find that you will do 2 or 3 sets for every 1 set that the people around you complete, because they rest between sets. You'll keep the routine to 30 minutes, with a goal of seeing how much energy you can expend in that time frame. You will be in perpetual motion. This is the difference between flying through life with a sense of direction and meandering through life like a goalie, fending off shots.

Strength training will increase your lean body mass, which is the key to a healthy physique. After the age of 25, we lose a pound of lean body mass each year unless we do something about it. For each pound of extra lean body mass you have, you burn an extra 50 calories a day. Even when you sleep, you'll burn more calories.

It's the difference between having a four-cylinder or an eight-cylinder engine. The eight-cylinder is going burn more fuel. Sure, it requires more fuel, but as we established in the Core Nutrition program, a hot fire burns more fuel. You'll be eating more often and fueling your body with nothing but the equivalent of high-test gasoline.

We've set up this program to ease you into the circuit training program. At the start of the program, you won't do any strength exercises at all. You'll never do more than six exercises, all progressing at a gradual pace. Once you've experienced the benefits of Movement Prep and Prehab, you'll have the foundation to perform the Strength regimen at maximum capacity. If you're pressed for time, do only Movement Prep and Prehab and find some time in your day for cardio exercise—for example, taking the stairs instead of the elevator at work—and you'll be fine.

Even though the strength workout is not aerobic exercise, you will get some aerobic benefit from the workout since your heart rate will increase and never fall below a certain aerobic zone. It's as if you're getting an aerobic workout, a two-for-one bonus. It's another example of how you will get the maximum benefit out of your 30 minutes.

By building strength and lean body mass through circuit training, you'll elevate your metabolism, and that elevated rate will last for *a few days,* as opposed to low-level cardiovascular training, which only gives the metabolism a short-term burst while exercising and in the hours immediately afterward.

One of the goals of this program is to increase work capacity, which is another measure of fitness. This is sometimes referred to as work density—a measure of how much work gets done per unit time. If I gave you X units' worth of work and it took you 30 minutes to accomplish today, with practice, it might only take 15 minutes 3 weeks later. Thus, you can accomplish more during that 30-minute period.

Your ability to perform in Level 4 will be the best indication of your current fitness. If you ever get knocked off of your Core program, you can figure out when you are back to your best by working back up to the level and stage you left off with, and then progressing from there.

That's a concrete way to measure increased fitness: more quality and quantity in less time. It's a lot like broadband versus a dial-up connection. You can measure progress in terms of time, number of repetitions, amount of weight used, and the number of times you can complete the circuit. If for some reason you miss a few workouts—or even a few weeks—you'll be able to measure the regression by discovering just how much you can get done in 30 minutes, and how it compares with your results before you fell off the program.

Strength training in the Core program is not just about increasing the strength of your larger muscles. It improves *stabilizing* strength, which supports proper alignment, movement patterns, and energy transfer and helps to reduces injuries. In short, the Strength unit acts as a foundation for all movement. The strength exercises we've selected are designed to increase your stabilizing strength most efficiently, and after we direct you to work on one movement, we've built in enough time to allow that area to recover while you work on something else. We'll start with an exercise that's an "upper-body push," such as pushups or an alternating dumbbell press. From there, we'll proceed to a "lower-body pull," then to an "upper-body pull" and a "lower-body push," all in a circuit fashion. We'll tie it all together with additional core work and multiplane rotational movements.

The Core Strength circuit increases the number of muscles being recruited throughout different parts of the body, to optimize your bloodflow and release positive hormones. By alternating exercises like this, you'll be able to do a few more reps each time or use a little more weight, and all in a shorter period of time. As a result, you'll increase the workout density—the quality and quantity of work per unit of time—improve your overall fitness, and enjoy cardiovascular benefits while increasing your balance, flexibility, stability, and mobility.

CARDIO (A.K.A. ENERGY-SYSTEM DEVELOPMENT)

Cardio work is perhaps the most misunderstood and most debated element of fitness. Some believe that it's unnecessary and prefer to focus exclusively on resistance training. Others misinterpret cardio training as a slog, which provides little return per investment of time. Whatever the case, I'm not a big fan of the term *cardio* because it's come to represent long, slow, sloppy movement. For most people, it means going out for a jog at the same steady pace for an hour, employing poor, inefficient movement patterns. For others, it entails hopping on a stationary bike, stairclimber, or treadmill for a steady but hardly strenuous 45 minutes.

This, obviously, does not provide a high return on your investment of time, and it goes against everything you're trying to accomplish with *Core Performance Essentials.* We want you to get more out of your 30 minutes on Tuesdays and Thursdays than others do who maintain a leisurely, undemanding pace.

Because of circuit training, you're already

INCREASE YOUR HORSEPOWER

In the world of thoroughbred racing, interval training is controversial. Owners of million-dollar horses do not want to risk injury by having the animals pushed through interval training. Unless the training is carefully monitored, it's possible that a horse's legs could buckle during the work interval.

Rather than take that risk, many owners prefer to rely on the horse's superior genetics and traditional training methods, which are the equine equivalent of going on a long, slow run or spending 30 leisurely minutes on a piece of gym equipment.

In many cases, that's sufficient. But there have been instances of $10,000 horses undergoing interval training and outracing million-dollar opponents. That's not a bad metaphor for the Core Essentials program. After all, the successful person is the one that departs from the pack to try something different, who relies not on natural gifts but on hard work and the will to constantly improve.

Unlike a thoroughbred horse, we don't have the advantage of being bred for physical performance. But by undergoing interval training, we can greatly increase our horsepower.

benefiting from a degree of cardio work. If you're making progress and increasing your workload, perhaps monitoring it with a pedometer or Adidas MOVE shoes, you're going to achieve a phenomenal cardio result. Don't feel bad if you don't have time for cardio on Tuesdays and Thursdays, because even without it, you're achieving results.

But just as you're investing the 30 minutes, 3 days a week, you'll get a phenomenal return on investment if you add 30 minutes of cardio, 2 days a week in Level 1. You might find that it helps you stick with your daily workout ritual and that it enables you to expend more calories by getting your body and mind moving.

Since this program is all about progression, I prefer to use terms such as *interval training* or Energy System Development. But since *cardio* is

so universally used, we'll stick with it here, recognizing that we're going to redefine the term.

Cardio is more than the 30 minutes you'll spend on Tuesdays and Thursdays. For starters, I want you to lead a more active lifestyle. Take the stairs instead of the elevator. Instead of circling the parking lot for the closest spot, park in the first one that's available. Ride a bike wherever you can, and even to work, if possible. Take the dog for a walk. Instead of sitting around watching your kid's soccer practice, walk around the field a few times, keeping an eye on the action.

Look for opportunities to move and exert energy. Avoid elevators. Walk, don't ride, escalators. Walk briskly alongside those moving sidewalks at the airport. Otherwise, you'll probably get stuck behind someone riding the sidewalk. (And there's that obesity epidemic again!) Life is one big *Buns of Steel* workout, right? Take advantage of the dozens of opportunities in front of you every day.

In Levels 2, 3, and 4, you'll be ready to take 1 of the 2 days and mix in some light "intervals"—periods of moderate exercise alternated with intense periods. With intervals, there will be times when I want you to work harder. Drop the conversation with your friends in the gym for a few moments, focus on working harder, and your heart rate will elevate. If you're out walking, try a light jog for 30 seconds to a couple of minutes, and then slow once more to a walk. Try and incorporate four to eight intervals during the course of your half-hour walk.

Intensity is far more important than volume. You're going to maintain the same volume—12 to 30 minutes—throughout the program, but you'll ratchet up the intensity as you go along.

The smaller the ratio of work to rest, the more you will improve your body's *lactate threshold*—its capacity to do high-intensity work. With anaerobic exercise, the body relies more on energy stores than it does on oxygen. It puts you in oxygen debt, which increases the burning sensation in muscles and makes the body compensate to get your heart rate to come back down.

But there's tremendous benefit to this. It's like a tuning a high-performance engine—in this case, the lungs, heart, and related systems. Interval training increases energy production in every cell and in the highways to those cells, allowing you to burn energy more efficiently.

With most cardio work, people believe that they're exercising much harder than they really are. Some gyms have "perceived exertion charts" on the wall where people can attach a number figure to how they feel. Most people go by sweat, which often is a function of how long they've been on the machine (if not the temperature in the room) and not how hard they've been working.

Gym equipment provides an effective cardio workout. Jump aboard a bike, treadmill, elliptical trainer, or Versaclimber. Set it on manual. Many of these machines are equipped with heart rate monitors. You grasp the handles, and within seconds the machine gives you a reading. But just because they're appropriate for the task, don't feel limited to gym machines. (Heart rate monitors are inexpensive, informative tools.) If you'd rather do your cardio work by attacking hills, biking, or even swimming, then by all means go for it. You could climb stairs or run a daunting hill in your neighborhood. Maybe there's a route that has a series of hills and flat surfaces. Wherever you choose to do your Cardio work, by following the *Core Performance Essentials* Workout you'll enjoy a cardio benefit, although it's important to do something else. Be active throughout the day and try to get in your 30 minutes of cardio.

It's never too early or too late to start. According to a recent study supported by the National Heart, Lung, and Blood Institute

(NHLBI), which is part of the National Institutes of Health, cardio-respiratory fitness in early adulthood significantly decreases the chance of developing high blood pressure and diabetes, which are both major risk factors for heart disease and stroke.

That's no surprise, of course. But the key is to maximize your effort with proper movement patterns through cardio work, not just to make the most of your time but also to safeguard your health, now and for the future.

The Cardio routine evolves in each of the four levels and stages. Each one starts with a warmup period of 3 minutes and a cooldown period ranging from 3 to 5 minutes, which will take you up to 30 minutes for each workout.

Cardio is no time to get sloppy with movement patterns. Regardless of the activity, you should feel tall and stabilized through your pillar. Focus on keeping both feet pointing straight ahead. Fire your glutes and quads, and don't forget to use your arms. You will be amazed at how much more fluid you feel, and at the amount of speed you can maintain with less effort.

In Level 1, we will focus on steady-state aerobic work. *Aerobic* simply means that your body will use oxygen to provide a steady and consistent, low level of energy for a long time, without building up any waste products in the body that hinder performance.

Think of it as a low-horsepower, highly fuel-efficient, four-cylinder engine that can run all day but does not generate a whole lot of power. A good rule of thumb for Level 1 is that you should be able to carry on a conversation when you are in the aerobic zone.

Some of the best activities for Level 1 are:

- Outdoors: Brisk walking, walking up hills, biking, swimming, rowing

- Indoors on cardio equipment: Biking, treadmill climbing/walking, elliptical trainer, Airdyne

Using the aerobic zone during Level 1 will improve your cardiovascular system and prepare your muscles for the greater speeds of Levels 2 through 4. This lower-level work will let your movement patterns, muscles, and joints adapt and prepare for the more intense training coming in these next phases.

When we get into Levels 2, 3, and 4, we will introduce interval training, where there will be bouts of harder effort mixed with easier-effort periods to give your body time to recover. We will use the lower-intensity Level 1 aerobic work in Levels 2 through 4—the more advanced zones of the program—as the recovery tool.

As with the Core Strength unit, interval training increases your body's release of positive hormones, which builds lean body mass and signals your body to dump fat. At the same time, it keeps your heart rate from dropping out of the aerobic zone.

Level 2 will introduce interval training by mixing moderate intensity with bouts of Level 1 easy-intensity aerobic work to allow you to catch your breath and recover from the slightly more intense intervals.

You will notice that these exercises include some work and some rest; we call this the work-to-rest ratio. The greater the rest, the higher quality the work should be. The lower the ratio—for instance, 1 second of rest per 1 second of work (one-to-one)—the bigger the challenge, since the body has less time to recover. That increases your capacity to do work.

You'll know you've reached Level 2 moderate intensity if you would find it difficult to carry on a conversation. You could, but you wouldn't be able to say much more than a couple of words at a time.

Some of the best activities for Level 2 are:

● Outdoors: Running-to-jogging/walking, jogging-to-walking

● Indoors: Bike, elliptical trainer, treadmill, stairclimbers, Airdyne

In Level 3, you will work harder. We are going to decrease the times and increase the rest intervals. Don't be intimidated by more intense work; you'll be ready for it. In fact, you will be looking for a greater challenge.

That brings us to Level 4, the shortest of the intervals. It's going to require you to use all of this newfound mobility, stability, and strength. At this level you will run, ride, or climb as hard as possible for between 10 and 30 seconds. In order to get the most out of Level 4, you'll need to pack as much power and energy into these segments as possible.

Some of the best activities for Level 4 are:

● Sprinting (flat or uphill)

● Shuttle runs (5 yards and back, 10 yards and back, 15 yards and back)

● Bicycle intervals

● Versaclimber sprints

The bottom line with the Core Cardio unit is that instead of slow, plodding workouts, we want to create a process where your muscles, nervous system, and hormones act together into efficient movement patterns and help your body work as efficiently as possible.

Chapter 9 Summary: The Core Workout is an integrated program that trains the body for lifelong movement. It consists of four components: Movement Preparation, Prehab, Strength, and Cardio. Movement Prep increases core temperature and lengthens and strengthens muscles so that you make long-term flexibility and stability gains. Prehab is the proactive approach to protecting yourself from injury by building "pillar strength," the integration of shoulder, trunk, and hip stability. Your body needs strength to sustain movement and everyday demands. We will improve the strength of the movements you were born with. Unlike traditional cardio work, the Core Cardio unit focuses on quality, not quantity, and it improves the function of your cardiovascular system while building endurance and helping your body create new energy levels.

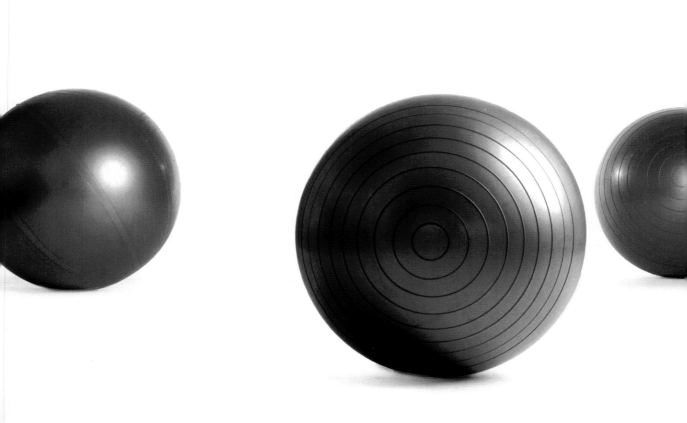

CHAPTER 10

CORE MOVEMENTS

I n 2005, the Department of Health and Human Services issued new guidelines to combat the nation's growing weight problem. It recommended that adults do about 60 minutes of "moderate to vigorous" physical activity daily to prevent weight gain. For those trying to maintain weight loss, they recommended 60 to 90 minutes. Previous guidelines called for just 30 minutes a day—and just one-third of adults reached that goal. So I'm guessing that with the bar raised, the percentages will get even worse. The problem with these recommendations is that they assume people work out at a meandering pace, if at all, and never push themselves.

All I want you to start with is exercise 3 days a week (Monday, Wednesday, and Friday) for 30 minutes at a time. If you have time to do some cardio work on Tuesdays and Thursdays, then make the most of those additional 30-minute intervals.

Anyone can find 30 minutes, 3 days a week, to make this small investment in his life. That's just 1.3 percent of your waking hours, assuming 8 hours of sleep a night. If you can make that commitment, I guarantee that the return on your investment will be exponential.

No matter how busy you are, you can find 30 minutes. Turn off the television—or at least set the VCR or TiVo. Get up earlier. Instead of going out to lunch, take advantage of that health club in your office. Schedule your workouts on a day planner or BlackBerry. That way, they'll become a core component of your lifestyle.

The upside is tremendous. Not only will you feel and look better, but you'll also create a body that's resistant to injury, long-term deterioration, and excruciating back pain. By following this program, in conjunction with Core Nutrition, you will build long-term health, not just temporary muscles for show.

Isn't it amazing that people take better care of their cars than of their bodies? They pay for the 3,000-mile oil changes and 30,000-mile checkup. They rotate the tires and change all of the filters and belts, all with the hope of getting maximum performance and the longest possible lifespan out of a vehicle unlikely to last more than 10 years, no matter how well they take care of it.

Why not take the same approach with your body? After all, you can always buy a new car, but your body you can't replace. Money and extended warranties can cure most any automotive problem. That's not the case with your health.

Speaking of money, think of how diligent people are when it comes to preparing for middle age and retirement: They make short-term sacrifices in order to properly finance college funds, retirement accounts, and other investments so that they can enjoy their golden years in comfort.

But what good is financial security if you're sick or confined to a wheelchair during your retirement? What good is financial security if you're lost to a stroke or heart attack? Taking just 90 minutes a week is a far smaller sacrifice than the ones you're probably already making for your financial future. Unlike financial planning, with its degree of uncertainty and risk, you know you'll get a return from this investment. Make this modest investment now and you can remain active well into your seventies, eighties, and nineties, improving the quality of your life.

With this program, we've eliminated all excuses. If you can't make it to a gym, we've provided exercise variations that can be done with nothing more than a mini band, a physioball, and a pair of dumbbells at home. If you're on the road or have no access to equipment, we've included versions that require nothing at all.

But wait, you say, it will take some time to get up to speed with the program. You've never done anything like this before. If that's the case, stop after 30 minutes. That's right. Call it a day. Pat yourself on the back. You'll find that as you master the movements, you can do the workout faster and thus get through more of it.

Our goal is not to create longer workouts but to pack more into our limited time. If you're already working out, you will have to think of your routines differently. You're not going to rest between sets or alternate exercises with a partner. Instead, you'll train opposite sets of movements, which is to say movements that tax different muscle groups, in circuits so that you don't need to stop. Work with your partner at the same time. By maintaining this pace, you'll find that *Core Performance Essentials* is a cardio workout in itself.

Since you're no doubt accustomed to multitasking in other areas of life, this should not be too much of an adjustment. Don't confuse this with talking on the cell phone or conducting business while working out. That's counterproductive—and disrespectful to the people on the other line and those around you at the gym. Make this a time for yourself.

If you think this workout is too easy, add sets, reps, or exercises to the Core Workout. Perform the advanced routines. Your progress is unlimited, though time is not. If you haven't tried my first book, *Core Performance,* you might want to give it a shot.

The reason most people spend so much time in the gym—or think that it's necessary— is because they never improve their work density. They add more reps, sets, and exercises, but because they work at a slow, plodding pace, it takes more time. We're not going to do that.

Have you ever prepared to give a speech or talk? If so, you've probably noticed that the more you practice, the shorter the talk becomes. It's not necessarily because you're talking faster or truncating parts, but you're becoming more comfortable with what you're saying. You might find that you can pack more into that 30-minute talk than you thought.

That's the same philosophy as with this workout. As you get more comfortable, you work more efficiently.

I've divided the Core Workout into four levels, which fall into three color zones: Red, Yellow, and Green. Think of it as a traffic light. Red means *stopping* your *inactivity.* If your body is tight, in pain, or out of shape, that's going to stop right here. You fall into the Red category if:

● You're really out of shape, meaning you haven't worked out in years—or ever.

● You're coming off of an injury-related layoff.

● You get some exercise, but your body is very tight—for instance, if you can't remember the last time you touched your toes.

● You used to work out regularly but, because of added time constraints, you haven't been doing much in recent months or years.

As with a traffic light, you should use caution in the Level 2 Yellow Zone. You've loosened up your body and have made great strides in the

Red Zone, but you're not quite ready for the full-blown Green Zone.

Marketing—"no pain, no gain"—has taught us that if we want to look like bodybuilders or fitness or fashion models, we must undergo daily suffering. When we don't achieve those results, despite Herculean efforts, we feel inadequate and disappointed. Workout programs fail not because people lack the effort but because they grind themselves down by doing more miles or repetitions until they have punished their bodies into submission.

Instead of falling into that pattern, stop while you're ahead. That way, when you come back for more, you'll be ready to achieve an even higher level of performance. Don't get me wrong; this program will help you look noticeably different in 3 short weeks. But you'll accomplish it the right way, with a view to the long run, to make sure you feel and perform better. The bottom line is that we need to shift our mindsets by understanding this new paradigm with these three main goals:

1. Decreasing pain (Red Zone—Level 1)

2. Preventing pain (Yellow Zone—Level 2)

3. Performing (Green Zone—Levels 3 and 4)

This traffic light analogy applies to training and to many other aspects of life. Before we are able to move forward in terms of our bodies, relationships, or finances, we must stop the downward spiral. We must decrease physi-

cal pain to enjoy the quality of life we deserve. Once the pain is diminished, we're free to exercise with the intent of regaining that lost function and "prehab" to make sure it does not happen again.

Think of this as the agility to quickly change directions in life. This is the line in the sand where you stop going in the wrong direction. Take an athlete cutting as an analogy. He is heading one way, then he stops and explodes to another direction, sprinting for his goal of scoring again.

It takes less-conditioned athletes longer to make this cut; some would call them slow. Highly conditioned athletes do it almost instantaneously, all game long. To be great athletes in the Game of Life, we have to do this several times per hour, as the tacklers (stress and chaos) force us to redirect ourselves and immediately continue on toward our core values and goals.

The Core Workout is organized into four levels or "zones":

Level 1

In football, teams like to be in the "red zone," because it means they're within 20 yards of the end zone. It's an exciting place to be, and that's the case with our Red Zone, also known as Level 1 of the Core Workout. This level will be the springboard to your success.

You're in the Red Zone because of pain that's keeping you from leading the quality of life you deserve. You have less energy and motivation to exercise, since it causes more pain. It is a degenerating and depressing free fall.

You will go through this pain at some point in your life if you don't take action. Maybe you're there already. We don't know what the Game of Life will throw at us, but we can take action now to prevent the decline. It all starts with getting out of the Red Zone and scoring touchdowns in real life.

Level 2

When you see a yellow light, you think "caution." Maybe you floor the gas pedal and speed through the light, or perhaps you come to a stop. It depends mostly on your position at the moment.

In our Yellow Zone, Level 2, we're exercising caution to make sure that we prevent injuries down the road. We can actually prevent more than 65 percent of injuries in sports and everyday life. We also can do a better job of preparing for and protecting ourselves from the severity of the remaining 35 percent of injuries, which are caused by traumatic events.

In the Yellow Zone of the Core Workout, we will focus on how to protect the most vulnerable areas of the body, making sure that everything is aligned and working in harmony. That way, there will be no excessive wear and tear caused by poor movement patterns. An ounce of prevention goes a very long way in life.

Levels 3 and 4

Now that you have taken the time to restore your body and protect it from injury, you will feel the desire to use it. By applying this energy in the right ways, you will fly down the performance highway.

As you enter the highway, you have to pick an on-ramp and start building up speed toward your destination, and that's exactly what you will do here. As you master and progress through Levels 3 and 4 of the Core Performance Essentials system, you will be able to merge with other high-performance vehicles through my first book, *Core Performance,* or better yet, through a version that's customized for you at www.coreperformance.com.

You will never be overly challenged, nor will you ever be bored to death and stifled by doing the same old thing. Being part of the Core community ensures your progress and evolution with convenient, fun, and affordable alternatives.

The Core Movement program will use these three goals—decreasing pain (Level 1, the Red Zone), preventing pain (Level 2, the Yellow Zone), and performing (Levels 3 and 4, the Green Zone)—from the very first Level 1 program to the highest levels of performance that the most elite athletes achieve during their career with Athletes' Performance.

Now let's take a look at how we're going to progress through the exercises. First, I want you to achieve and experience some success. After that, I will be honored to gradually challenge you more and more until you look back one day and shake your head in disbelief over how far you have come.

The Surgeon General asked everyone to exercise 60 minutes, five or six times a week. Let's get you moving in that direction by cutting that in half and focus on achieving the highest return on your time investment. We will fire up this engine, and it will take on a life of its own because it will become part of *your* core.

In chapter 12, Quality of Time, you will be asked to block out a consistent 30 minutes a day, three times a week for your Core Routine, with a day in between for simple cardio and regeneration, which may be done all at once or throughout the day. (See chapter 11 for more on the concept of Regeneration.)

We have created a simple, progressive, four-level program that will keep you challenged for years.

You will begin each level with Stage A, requiring 1 set of 6 repetitions, building up to where you can go through part of this workout twice. As soon as you are able to perform these exercises properly in the allotted time, you will add 2 reps, for a total of 8. You will then repeat this process, and bump up 2 more, to 10 reps.

When you can go through the levels for the prescribed number of circuits per unit (Movement Prep, Prehab, Strength), and the desired number of reps with movement mastery, do something special for yourself. Compare notes with fellow Core participants. Celebrate victories in life and share them with your family and friends. You are then ready to move up to the next level.

LEVEL	STAGE A	STAGE B	STAGE C	STAGE D	TIME DISTRIBUTION
1	1 × 6	2 × 6	2 × 8	2 × 10	Movement Prep: 15 min Prehab: 15 min
2	1 × 6	2 × 6	2 × 8	2 × 10	Movement Prep: 10 min Prehab: 10 min Strength: 10 min
3	1 × 6	2 × 6	2 × 8	2 × 10	Movement Prep: 7 min Prehab: 8 min Strength: 15 min
4	1 × 6	2 × 6	2 × 8	2 × 10	Movement Prep: 7 min Prehab: 8 min Strength: 15 min

The next level will repeat the same process, but I have added an exercise to each unit and increased the complexity. I will increase the demands ever so slightly within each unit and each exercise by increasing the range of motion or the amount of stability, mobility, balance, or strength required. Or I might have decreased the amount of time allotted to complete the unit.

LEVEL 1: THE RED ZONE

Everyone starts here, with a 30-minute commitment, three times in Week One. Consider it your birth, indoctrination, or pregame warmup for the Core Routine. We're all rookies to the Core Routine, and just like every rookie in every other league, we too have to show up to training camp before the veterans. Even if you've done the *Core Performance* routine in the past, this will be a good refresher.

This runs parallel to the nutrition chapter, where we started by eating four healthy meals, 4 days a week. Here we will learn four exercises in Movement Prep and four exercises in Prehab. The goal of this workout is to take inventory of your body—right side versus left, front versus back, areas of tightness, balance, coordination, and strength. Next, you should perfect these movements and gain confidence by awakening all those long-dormant little muscles.

How long you stay at this level depends on several factors. If you are in fairly good shape and progressing easily, you might need only 1 week before moving on to Level 2. For example, you might do Stage A and find that you have plenty of time on the clock to do one more round of each unit, which is Stage B.

That may very well mean that you're ready to graduate to Stage C on Wednesday. Here you will add 2 reps to each exercise for 2 circuits each. On Friday, you will add 2 more reps for a total of 10 repetitions in Stage D. The following week, you will start on Level 2, Stage A, and you'll find out more about what's at your core.

If you're in pain or "deconditioned"—that is, if you're so tight that you haven't touched your toes since childhood, you have never trained before, or you've gone a long time since exercising—it might take 2 weeks to achieve mastery. Don't be alarmed if it takes longer than that. This will require patience, but think of it as turning on a car. When a car has been sitting in the garage, it takes more effort to get it started the first time. But once you do, it will come back to life quickly. Your body, likewise, will progress more rapidly from this point.

LEVEL 2: THE YELLOW ZONE

You now know the basics of the routine, but here I have added a few levels to each exercise and made the Movement Prep and Prehab routines more complex, while decreasing the time to 10 minutes for each unit. I have also added a third unit: Strength. You now have three units of five exercises, with 10 minutes to complete each unit.

In Level 2, you have to start slow and gradually build up speed and proficiency. To make sure that you achieve gains in strength, flexibility, and stability from the first workout, you will go through each unit only once, for a total of 1 set of 6 repetitions per exercise.

The goal is to formally start your training process. Here you are working on rehabbing to alleviate the discomfort you already feel and prehabbing to prevent future pain and dysfunction. This Level 2 workout will be your benchmark. If for whatever reason you get knocked off your Core Routine, you will have the resiliency of that Super Ball and bounce back quickly; you will start again with Level 2, Stage A. You will then start working up the ladder with a progressive workout that evolves each session until you face an exciting and challenging routine. This will be your baseline.

Remember that you have only 30 minutes, divided equally into three 10-minute blocks. Keep an eye on the clock, and get as much done as you can in one unit. If you have gone through 1½ times, and the timer goes off,

stop; and move on to the next section. This is part of your challenge, decreasing your rest intervals and increasing the reps as you become more fit.

You will graduate from this level when you complete Stage D for 2 circuits, doing 10 perfect repetitions each, within 30 minutes.

LEVEL 3: THE GREEN ZONE

Green means go. You are starting to get in shape. Now that you're really on the road to increased performance, let's take things up a notch.

The theme here is "getting superstable." I am going to challenge you in Movement Prep, first by adding another exercise, but also by having you start covering ground with every rep, which will require more balance, stability, mobility, and strength.

In Prehab, there's another new exercise, taking you up to six. We'll also increase the complexity of your stabilizing strength with more "rotary" stability, working those ever-important rotator cuffs.

The Strength circuit is also cranked up a notch by incorporating the physioball to increase the stability challenge. This will result in increased muscle recruitment and total body integration. The goal is to minimize ball movement. You might notice your body and the ball shaking—your body is trying to gain neuromuscular control by firing more often to control the unstable surface. I like to call this wasted movement and energy "noise." Your aim, then, is to become more efficient and silence the "noise" by improving your ability to stabilize your body.

If you need others for motivation, have your training partner—whether they're with you or across the country and available only via phone or www.coreperformance.com—set the date, and go head-to-head to motivate and help each other reach new heights.

You'll note that you barely need dumbbells in Level 3. That's by design. Our goal with this unit is to stabilize our bodies, and we can do that with minimal weights. Not only that, but sometimes you're traveling or don't have access to dumbbells and need a no-equipment regimen.

LEVEL 4

In Level 4, we take things up yet another notch, with dumbbells to build strength. We're still in the Green Zone, only now we're going to challenge our bodies further. There might be times when you won't have access to dumbbells. When that's the case, stick with Level 3.

Chapter 10 Summary: In just 30 minutes a day, you're going to change your body and your mindset about working out. You'll do this by achieving three goals: decreasing pain, preventing pain, and performing at a high level. You'll progress through three workout zones: Red, Yellow, and Green. As you advance, the idea is not to spend more time working out but to make the most of that 30 minutes, creating greater "work density." Unlike other workout regimens, the Core Workout features unlimited progressions.

LEVEL 1: GET READY

MOVEMENT PREP (15 MINUTES)

STAGE:	A	B	C	D
NO. OF CIRCUITS:	1	2	2	2
REPETITIONS:	6 EA	6 EA	8 EA	10 EA

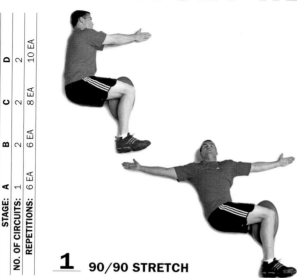

1 90/90 STRETCH

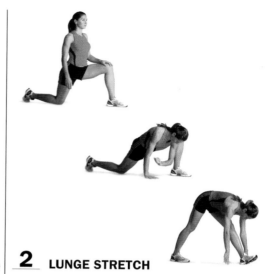

2 LUNGE STRETCH

PREHAB (15 MINUTES)

STAGE:	A	B	C	D
NO. OF CIRCUITS:	1	2	2	2
REPETITIONS:	6 EA	6 EA	8 EA	10 EA
OR TIME:	12 SEC	12 SEC	16 SEC	20 SEC

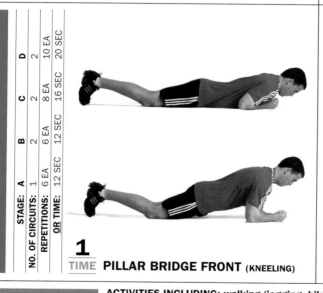

1 TIME PILLAR BRIDGE FRONT (KNEELING)

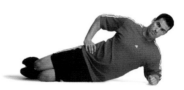
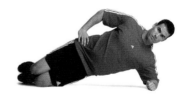

2 REPS PILLAR BRIDGE LATERAL (KNEELING)

CARDIO

ACTIVITIES INCLUDING: walking/jogging, biking, swimming; also, cardio equipment such as treadmill, stationary bike, or elliptical trainer.

STAGE:	A	B	C	D
WORK: (STEADY, LOW INTENSITY)	18 MIN	18 MIN	24 MIN	30 MIN

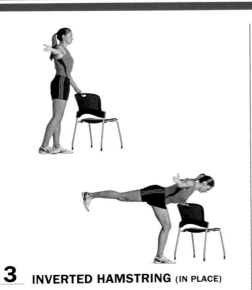

3 INVERTED HAMSTRING (IN PLACE)

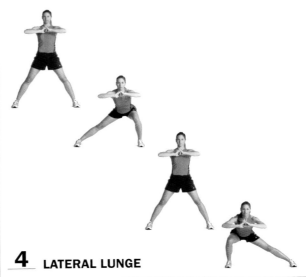

4 LATERAL LUNGE

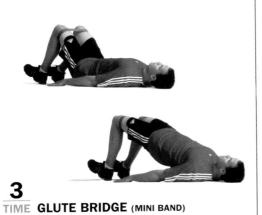

3 TIME GLUTE BRIDGE (MINI BAND)

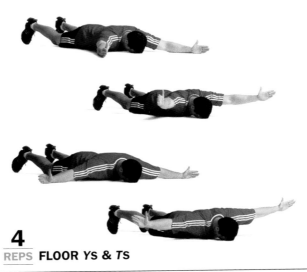

4 REPS FLOOR YS & TS

● Progress to the next <u>stage</u> when you successfully complete the prescribed number of circuits in the allotted time.

● Progress to the next <u>level</u> when you successfully complete Stage D with perfect technique in the desired time.

LEVEL 2: GET SET...GO!

MOVEMENT PREP (10 MINUTES)

STAGE:	A	B	C	D
NO. OF CIRCUITS:	1	1	1	1
REPETITIONS:	6 EA	6 EA	8 EA	10 EA

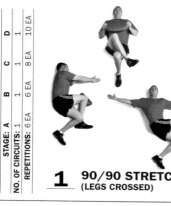

1 90/90 STRETCH (LEGS CROSSED)

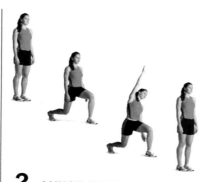

2 LUNGE STRETCH (BACKWARD)

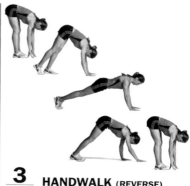

3 HANDWALK (REVERSE)

PREHAB (10 MINUTES)

STAGE:	A	B	C	D
NO. OF CIRCUITS:	1	2	2	2
REPETITIONS:	6 EA	6 EA	8 EA	10 EA
OR TIME:	12 SEC	12 SEC	16 SEC	20 SEC

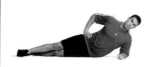
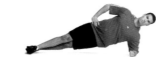

1 TIME — PILLAR BRIDGE FRONT

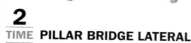

2 TIME — PILLAR BRIDGE LATERAL

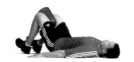
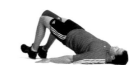

3 REPS — GLUTE BRIDGE (PADDED)

STRENGTH CIRCUIT (10 MINUTES)

STAGE:	A	B	C	D
NO. OF CIRCUITS:	1	2	2	2
REPETITIONS:	6 EA	6 EA	8 EA	10 EA

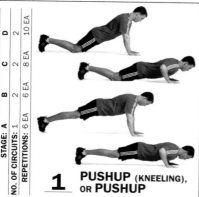

1 PUSHUP (KNEELING), OR PUSHUP

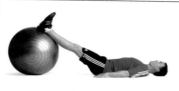
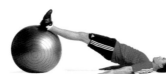

2 GLUTE BRIDGE (WITH PHYSIOBALL)

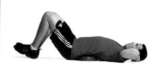
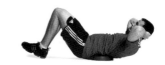

3 FLOOR CRUNCH (DOUBLE THE NUMBER OF REPS)

CARDIO

ACTIVITIES INCLUDING: walking/jogging, biking, swimming; also, cardio equipment such as treadmill, stationary bike, or elliptical trainer.

	A	B	C	D
WARMUP: 3 MINUTES				
STAGE:	A	B	C	D
WORK: (MODERATE)	1 MIN	1 MIN	2 MIN	3 MIN
RECOVERY: (EASY)	3 MIN	3 MIN	3 MIN	3 MIN
NO. OF REPS:	3X	4X	4X	3X
COOLDOWN: 5 MINUTES				
TOTAL TIME:	20 MIN	24 MIN	28 MIN	26 MIN

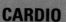

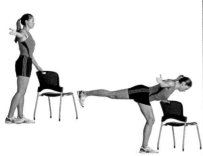

4 **INVERTED HAMSTRING**
(IN PLACE)

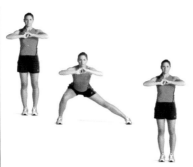

5 **LATERAL LUNGE**
(STEP AND RETURN)

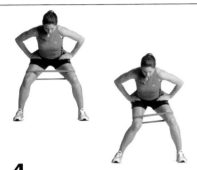

4
REPS **MINI BAND STANDING**

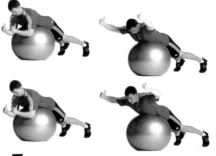

5
REPS **PHYSIOBALL** YS & TS
(ARMS BENT)

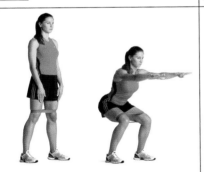

4 **SQUAT** (BODY WEIGHT,
WITH MINI BAND)

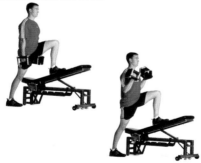

5 **SPLIT DUMBBELL CURL**

● Progress to the next <u>stage</u> when you successfully complete
the prescribed number of circuits in the allotted time.

● Progress to the next <u>level</u> when you successfully complete
Stage D with perfect technique in the desired time.

LEVEL 3: GET STABLE

MOVEMENT PREP (7 MINUTES)

STAGE:	A	B	C	D
NO. OF CIRCUITS:	1	1	1	1
REPETITIONS:	3 EA	3 EA	4 EA	5 EA

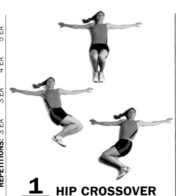

1 HIP CROSSOVER

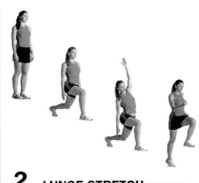

2 LUNGE STRETCH (MOVING)

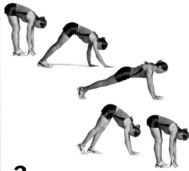

3 HANDWALK

PREHAB (8 MINUTES)

STAGE:	A	B	C	D
NO. OF CIRCUITS:	1	1	1	1
REPETITIONS:	6 EA	6 EA	8 EA	10 EA
OR TIME:	12 SEC	12 SEC	16 SEC	20 SEC

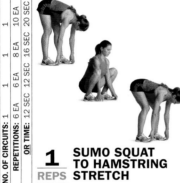

1 REPS **SUMO SQUAT TO HAMSTRING STRETCH**

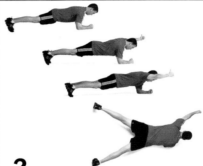

2 REPS **PILLAR BRIDGE FRONT** (WIDE FEET)

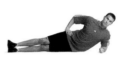

3 TIME **PILLAR BRIDGE LATERAL** (STACKED FEET)

STRENGTH CIRCUIT (15 MINUTES)

STAGE:	A	B	C	D
NO. OF CIRCUITS:	1	2	2	2
REPETITIONS:	6 EA	6 EA	8 EA	10 EA

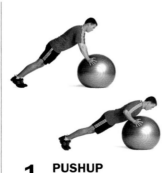

1 PUSHUP (WITH PHYSIOBALL)

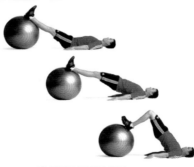

2 GLUTE BRIDGE (WITH PHYSIOBALL LEG CURL)

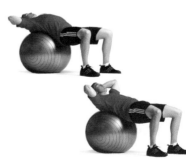

3 PHYSIOBALL CRUNCH (DOUBLE THE NUMBER OF REPS)

CARDIO

ACTIVITIES INCLUDING: walking/jogging, biking, swimming; also, cardio equipment such as treadmill, stationary bike, elliptical trainer, or Versaclimber.

	A	B	C	D
WARMUP: 3 MINUTES				
STAGE:	A	B	C	D
WORK: (HARD)	2 MIN	2 MIN	1 MIN	30 SEC
RECOVERY: (EASY)	2 MIN	2 MIN	1 MIN	30 SEC
NO. OF REPS:	3X	4X	6X	8X
COOLDOWN: 5 MINUTES				
TOTAL TIME:	20 MIN	24 MIN	20 MIN	16 MIN

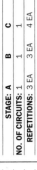
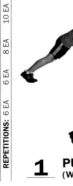

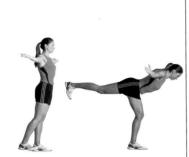

4 INVERTED HAMSTRING (BACKWARD)

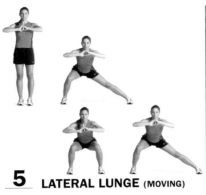

5 LATERAL LUNGE (MOVING)

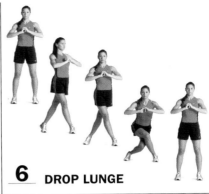

6 DROP LUNGE

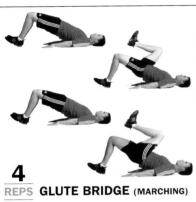

4 REPS GLUTE BRIDGE (MARCHING)

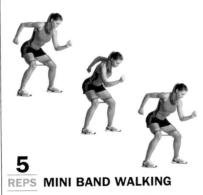

5 REPS MINI BAND WALKING

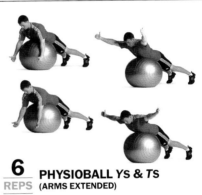

6 REPS PHYSIOBALL *Y*S & *T*S (ARMS EXTENDED)

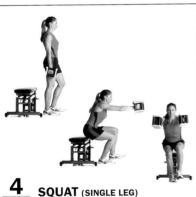

4 SQUAT (SINGLE LEG)

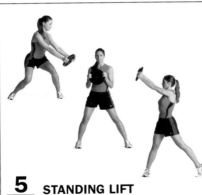

5 STANDING LIFT

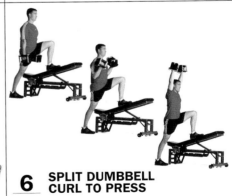

6 SPLIT DUMBBELL CURL TO PRESS

● Progress to the next <u>stage</u> when you successfully complete the prescribed number of circuits in the allotted time.

● Progress to the next <u>level</u> when you successfully complete Stage D with perfect technique in the desired time.

MOVEMENT PREP (7 MINUTES)

STAGE:	A	B	C	D
NO. OF CIRCUITS:	1	1	1	1
REPETITIONS:	5 EA	5 EA	4 EA	3 EA

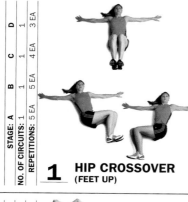

1 HIP CROSSOVER (FEET UP)

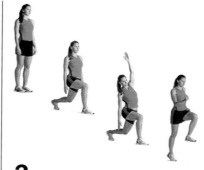

2 LUNGE STRETCH (MOVING)

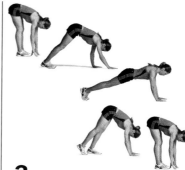

3 HANDWALK

PREHAB (8 MINUTES)

STAGE:	A	B	C	D
NO. OF CIRCUITS:	1	1	1	1
REPETITIONS:	6 EA	6 EA	8 EA	10 EA

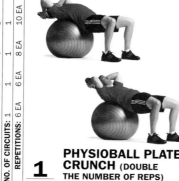

1 PHYSIOBALL PLATE CRUNCH (DOUBLE THE NUMBER OF REPS)

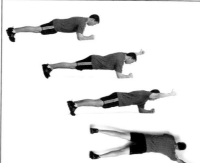

2 PILLAR BRIDGE FRONT (NARROW FEET)

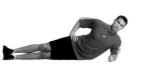
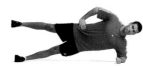

3 PILLAR BRIDGE LATERAL (JUMPING JACK)

STRENGTH CIRCUIT (15 MINUTES)

STAGE:	A	B	C	D
NO. OF CIRCUITS:	1	2	2	2
REPETITIONS:	6 EA	6 EA	8 EA	10 EA

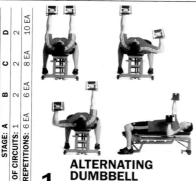

1 ALTERNATING DUMBBELL BENCH PRESS

2 ROMANIAN DEADLIFT (TWO ARMS, ONE LEG)

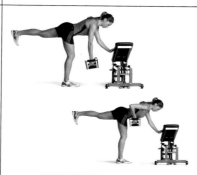

3 ONE-ARM, ONE-LEG DUMBBELL ROW

CARDIO

ACTIVITIES INCLUDING: walking/sprinting, biking, swimming; also, cardio equipment such as treadmill, stationary bike, or Versaclimber.

WARMUP: 3 MINUTES EASY CARDIO AND 3 MINUTES MOVEMENT PREP				
STAGE:	A	B	C	D
WORK: (VERY HARD)	10 SEC	15 SEC	20 SEC	30 SEC
RECOVERY: (EASY)	50 SEC	45 SEC	40 SEC	30 SEC
NO. OF REPS:	12X	12X	12X	12X
COOLDOWN: 5 MINUTES—MAKE SURE TO REGEN TONIGHT!				
TOTAL TIME:	23 MIN	23 MIN	23 MIN	23 MIN

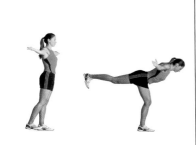

4 INVERTED HAMSTRING (BACKWARD)

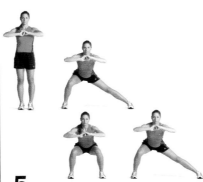

5 LATERAL LUNGE (MOVING)

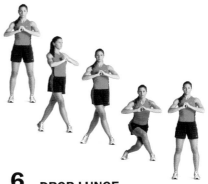

6 DROP LUNGE

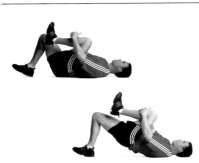

4 GLUTE BRIDGE (KNEE BENT)

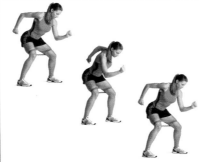

5 MINI BAND WALKING (ADD RESISTANCE)

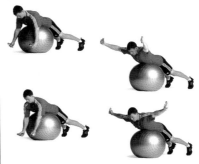

6 PHYSIOBALL YS & TS (WITH WEIGHT)

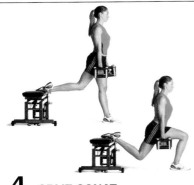

4 SPLIT SQUAT

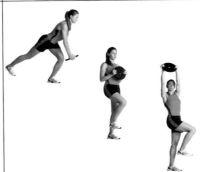

5 STANDING LIFT (ONE LEG)

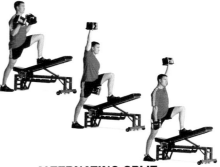

6 ALTERNATING SPLIT DUMBBELL CURL TO PRESS

● Progress to the next <u>stage</u> when you successfully complete the prescribed number of circuits in the allotted time.

● CONGRATULATIONS! Now progress to the next level by customizing your program at www.coreperformance.com.

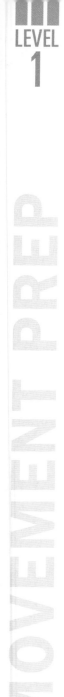

MOVEMENT PREP

90/90 STRETCH

PROCEDURE:

Lie on the ground on your left side in a fetal position, with your legs tucked up into your torso at a 90-degree angle and a pad or rolled-up towel between your knees. Keep both arms straight at a 90-degree angle to your torso. Now, keeping your knees together and on the ground and your hips still, rotate your chest and right arm back to the right, trying to put your back on the ground. Exhale and hold for 2 seconds, then return to the starting position. Finish your reps, then switch sides and repeat.

COACHING KEY:

Keep your knees together and pressed against the ground. Only rotate as far as you can without lifting or separating your knees. Exhale as you stretch.

YOU SHOULD FEEL:

A stretch through your torso and the muscles of your middle and upper back.

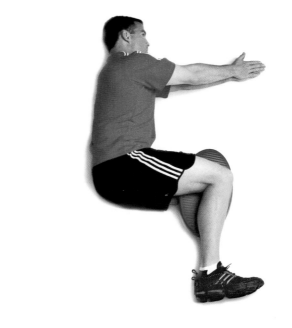

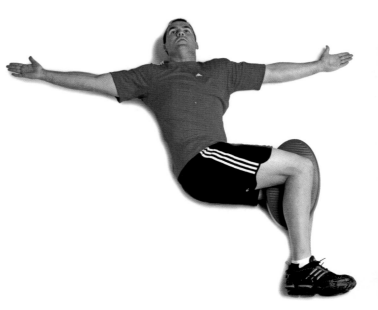

90/90 STRETCH (LEGS CROSSED)

PROCEDURE:

Lie faceup on the ground holding a pad or towel roll, your left knee bent to 90 degrees, and your right leg crossed over the left. Roll over onto your left side and pin a pad between your right knee and the ground. Maintaining pressure on the pad and keeping your hips still, rotate your chest and right arm back to the right, trying to put your back on the ground. Hold for 2 seconds, then return to the starting position. Repeat until you've completed your reps, then switch sides.

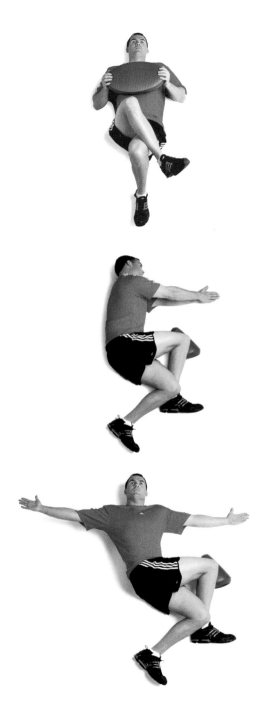

HIP CROSSOVER

PROCEDURE:

Lie faceup on the ground with your arms to your sides, your knees bent, and your feet flat. Twist your bent legs to the left until they reach the floor, then twist them to the right. Continue for the prescribed number of repetitions.

COACHING KEY:

Keep your shoulders on the ground, your knees together, and your stomach tight. Do not let your knees touch the ground.

YOU SHOULD FEEL:

A lengthening and strengthening of the torso.

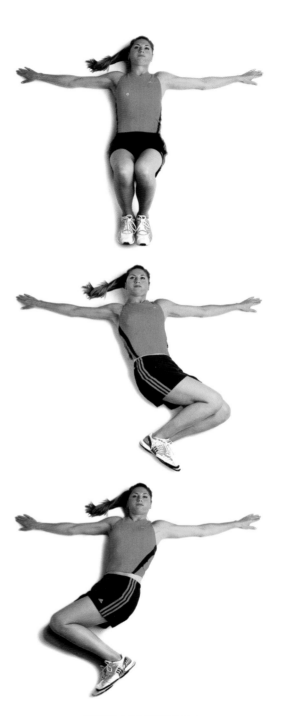

HIP CROSSOVER (FEET UP)

Try this move with your hips and knees bent 90 degrees and your feet off the ground. Once you master that, perform this move with your legs straight.

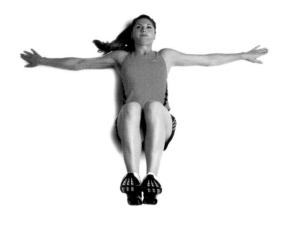

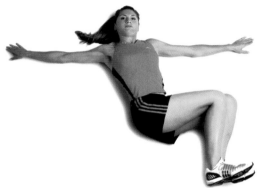

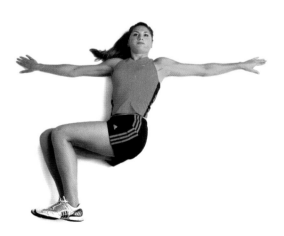

MOVEMENT PREP

LUNGE STRETCH

PROCEDURE:

Take a half-step forward with your left foot, placing your right hand on the floor for balance. Take your left elbow and reach down your instep (on your forward leg). Place your left hand on the floor and push your hips upward as you straighten your front leg. Return to the starting position and repeat.

COACHING KEY:

Contract (squeeze) the glute muscle of your back leg.

YOU SHOULD FEEL:

A stretch through the groin, the hip flexor muscle of your back leg, the glute muscle of your front leg, and your hamstring.

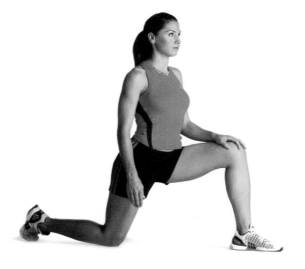

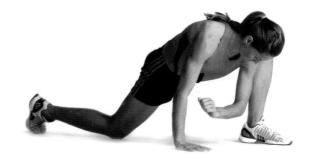

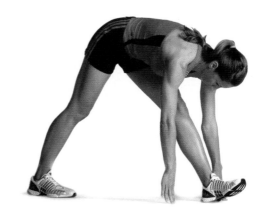

LUNGE STRETCH (BACKWARD)

PROCEDURE:

With your feet together, step back with your right leg into a lunge. While reaching your right hand to the sky, bend your torso to the left. Straighten your torso and step forward into the starting position. Alternate sides and repeat for the prescribed repetitions.

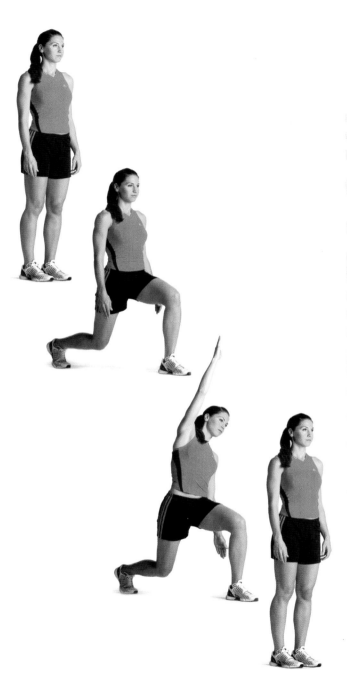

MOVEMENT PREP

LUNGE STRETCH (MOVING)

PROCEDURE:

Instead of returning to the starting position as in Level 2, walk forward into the next position.

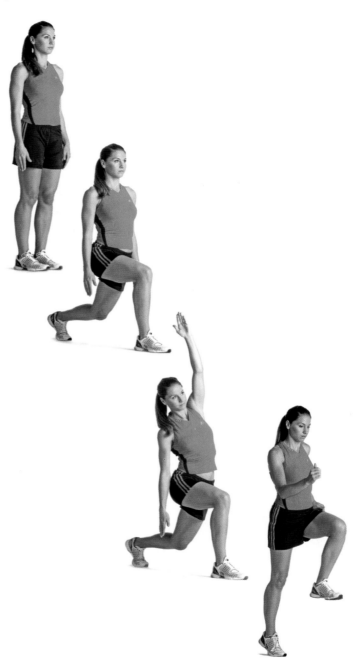

INVERTED HAMSTRING (IN PLACE)

PROCEDURE:

Stand on one leg with perfect posture, holding on to a wall, chair, or table for stability. Keep your shoulder blades back and down. Maintaining a straight line from ear to ankle, bend over at the waist, raising your opposite heel to the sky. When you feel a stretch, return to the standing position by contracting the muscles of your hamstring, glutes, and back. Complete your reps on that side, then switch legs.

COACHING KEY:

Keep your back flat and your hips and shoulders parallel to the ground. Maintain a straight line from your ear through your hip, knee, and ankle. Try to keep your balance without relying on your hand, and keep your opposite foot off the ground.

YOU SHOULD FEEL:

A stretch in your hamstrings.

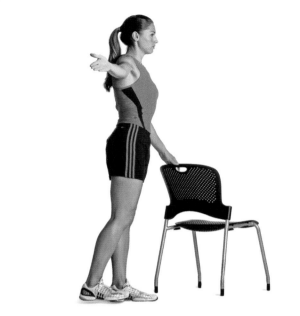

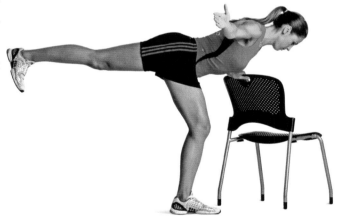

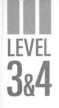

INVERTED HAMSTRING (BACKWARD)

PROCEDURE:

Step back into the next step and repeat using the opposite leg, alternating legs until you've completed all your reps.

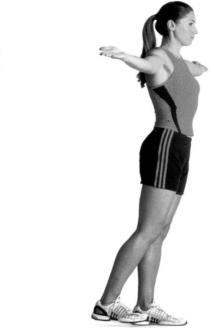

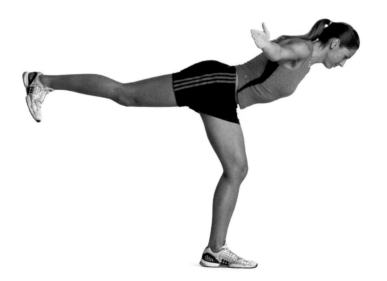

LATERAL LUNGE

PROCEDURE:

Standing with your feet wider than shoulder width apart, shift your hips to the left and down by bending your left knee and keeping your right leg straight. Your feet should be straight ahead and flat on the ground. Push through your left hip, returning to the starting position. Alternate sides and repeat for the prescribed number of repetitions.

COACHING KEY:

Keep your knee on your "working" side behind your toes. Keep your opposite leg straight, your back flat, and your chest up.

YOU SHOULD FEEL:

A lengthening and strengthening of your glutes, groin, hamstrings, and quads.

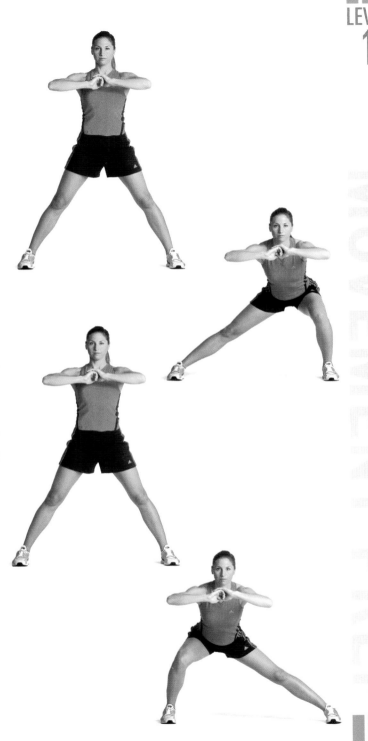

MOVEMENT PREP

LATERAL LUNGE (STEP AND RETURN)

PROCEDURE:

Step to the right with your right foot, keeping your toes forward and your feet flat. Squat through your right hip while keeping your left leg straight. Squat as low as possible, holding this position for 2 seconds. Push back to the starting position and repeat to the opposite side.

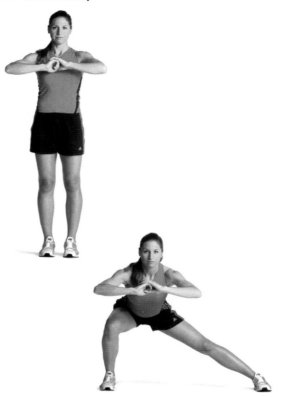

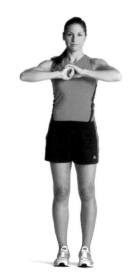

LATERAL LUNGE (MOVING)

PROCEDURE:

Instead of returning to the starting position, step into a squat position and then into the next lunge. Repeat for the prescribed number of repetitions and then switch sides. You will be stepping around the room during this exercise, so give yourself plenty of space.

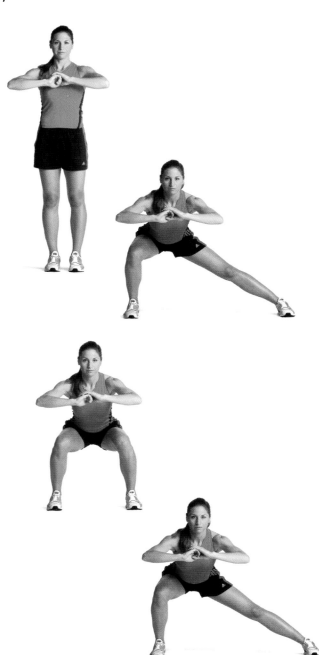

HANDWALK (REVERSE)

PROCEDURE:

Bend at the waist and walk your feet out into a pushup position. Now, keeping your knees straight, walk your hands toward your feet. When you feel a stretch, walk your feet back out to a pushup position. Repeat until you've completed your reps.

COACHING KEY:

Keep your knees straight and your stomach tight. Walk your hands out farther beyond your head for increased difficulty. Use short "ankle steps" to walk back up to your hands. That is, take baby steps using only your ankles—don't use your knees, hips, or quads.

YOU SHOULD FEEL:

A stretch in your hamstrings, lower back, glutes, and calves.

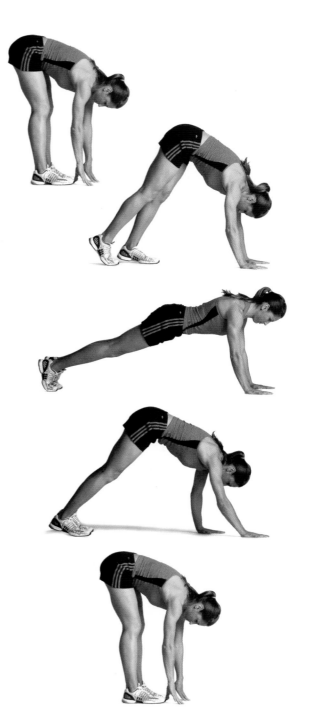

HANDWALK

PROCEDURE:

Instead of walking your feet back, walk your hands forward into a pushup position. Keeping your knees straight, walk your feet toward your hands until you feel a stretch in your hamstrings. Walk your hands forward to begin the next repetition. You will be moving around the rooms during this exercise, so give yourself plenty of space.

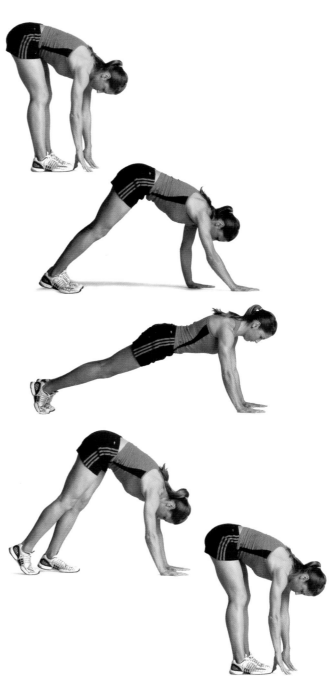

MOVEMENT PREP

MOVEMENT PREP

DROP LUNGE

PROCEDURE:

Reach your left foot 2 feet behind your right foot. Square your hips back to the starting position, and sit back and down into a squat. Stand and step laterally with your right foot, then repeat the stretch on the same side. Continue until you've completed your reps on that side, then reverse directions.

COACHING KEY:

Keep your chest up and sit your hips back. Maintain your weight on the heel of your front leg. You will be moving around the room during this exercise, so give yourself plenty of space.

YOU SHOULD FEEL:

A stretch in the outsides of both hips.

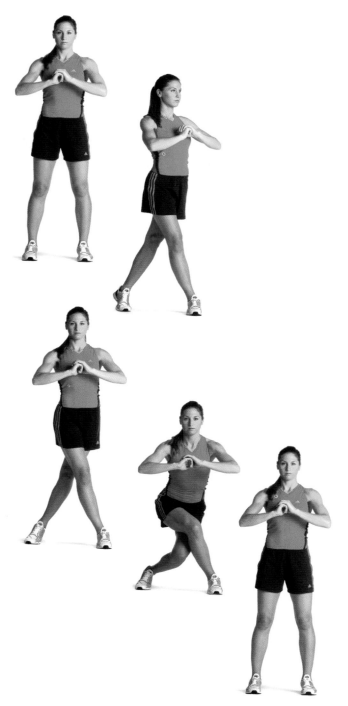

PILLAR BRIDGE FRONT (KNEELING)

PROCEDURE:

Lying on your stomach with your fore-arms on the ground under your chest, push off of your elbows, supporting your weight on your forearms and knees. Hold a static position for the prescribed length of time. Push your neck and sternum as far up and away from your forearms as possible.

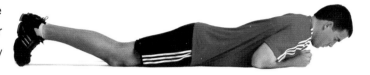

COACHING KEY:

Keep your stomach tight.

YOU SHOULD FEEL IT:

In your shoulders and trunk.

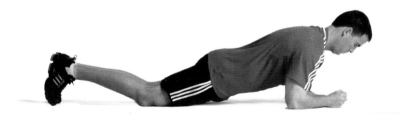

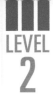
PILLAR BRIDGE FRONT

PROCEDURE:

Same procedure as for Level 1, but instead of finishing with your knees on the floor, end in a prone pushup position, with just your forearms and toes resting on the floor. Push your chest as far away from the ground as possible. Hold your position for the prescribed amount of time.

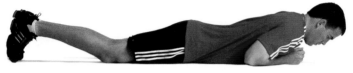

COACHING KEY:

Keep your tummy tight and your head in line with your spine. There should be a straight line between your ear and your ankle, with no sagging or bending.

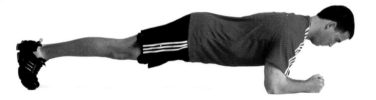

PILLAR BRIDGE FRONT (WIDE FEET)

PROCEDURE:

Lift one arm, hold for 2 seconds. Switch arms. Widen your feet, if necessary, to reduce difficulty.

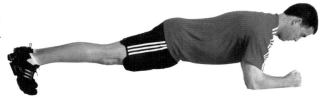

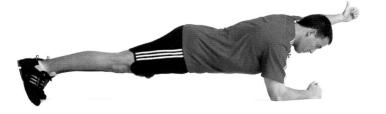

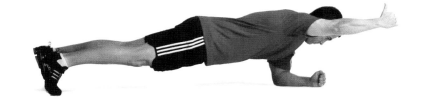

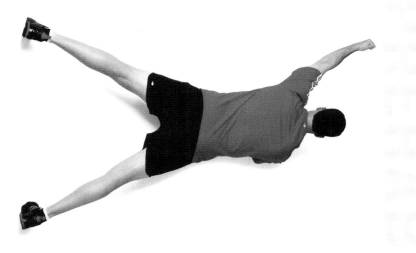

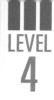

PILLAR BRIDGE FRONT (NARROW FEET)

PROCEDURE:

Same exercise as in Level 3. This time, narrow your feet to add to the degree of difficulty.

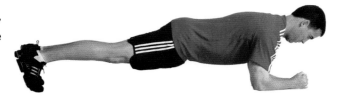

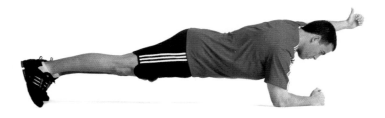

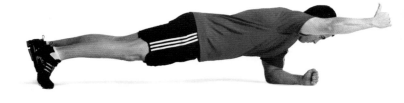

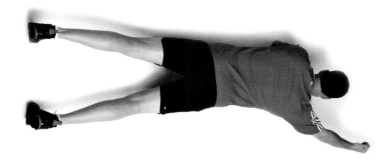

PILLAR BRIDGE LATERAL (KNEELING)

PROCEDURE:

Lie on your side with your forearm on the ground and your elbow under your shoulder, with your knees bent to 90 degrees. Push your forearm away from your body, lifting your hips into the air and supporting your weight on your forearm and knees. Hold a static position for the prescribed amount of time. Complete the reps on one side, then switch.

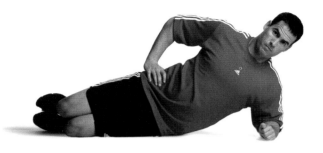

COACHING KEY:

Keep your body in a straight line and keep your stomach tight. If this is too difficult, do individual repetitions— 1 repetition per 2 seconds.

YOU SHOULD FEEL IT:

In your shoulders and trunk.

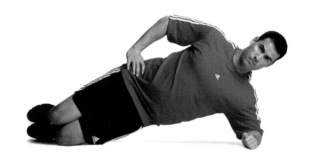

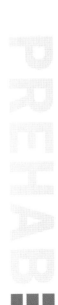
PREHAB

PILLAR BRIDGE LATERAL

PROCEDURE:

Lie on your side with your forearm on the ground under your shoulder, your feet split with the top leg forward. With your body in a straight line and your elbow under your shoulder, push your hip off the ground, creating a straight line from ankle to shoulder and keeping your head in line with your spine. Hold your position for the prescribed amount of time.

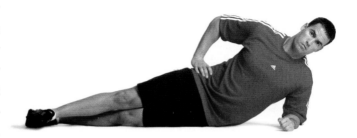

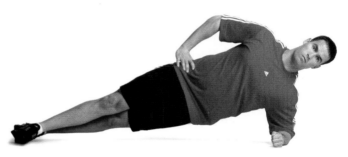

WWW.COREPERFORMANCE.COM

PILLAR BRIDGE LATERAL (STACKED FEET)

PROCEDURE:

Instead of splitting your feet, stack them together.

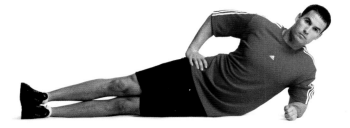

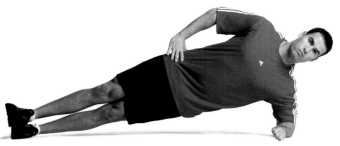

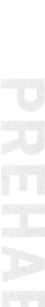

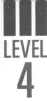

PILLAR BRIDGE LATERAL (JUMPING JACK)

PROCEDURE:

From the bridge position, lift your top leg into the air as if you were doing a lateral jumping jack.

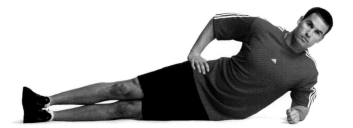

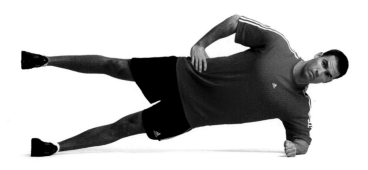

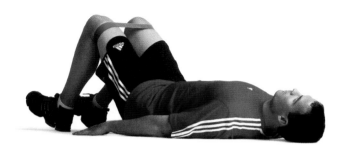
GLUTE BRIDGE (MINI BAND)

PROCEDURE:

Place a mini band just above your knees. Lying faceup on the ground with your arms to your sides, your knees bent, and your heels on the ground, lift your hips off the ground until your knees, hips, and shoulders are in a straight line. Hold for the prescribed time. If this is too difficult, divide the time into 2- to 3-second intervals, then return to the starting position and repeat until you've completed all of your prescribed time.

COACHING KEY:

Fire (squeeze) your glutes.

YOU SHOULD FEEL IT:

In your glutes, and to a lesser degree in your hamstrings and lower back.

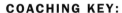

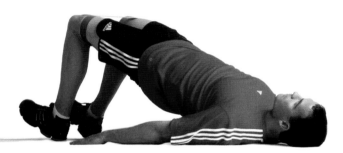

PREHAB

GLUTE BRIDGE (PADDED)

PROCEDURE:

Squeeze a rolled-up towel, a doubled-over Thera-Band pad, or even a ball between your knees. Lift your hips into the air and then return to the starting position. Repeat for the prescribed number of reps.

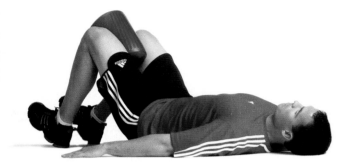

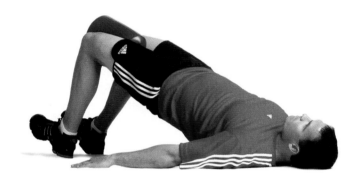

GLUTE BRIDGE (MARCHING)

PROCEDURE:

Try "marching" with one leg at a time.

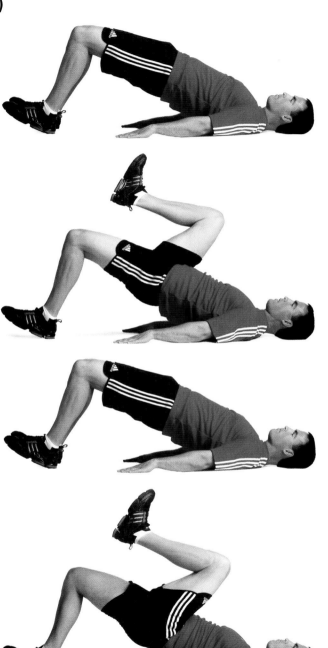

PREHAB

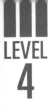

GLUTE BRIDGE (KNEE BENT)

PROCEDURE:

Try it with one leg held to your chest and your weight supported on the other leg. Switch legs.

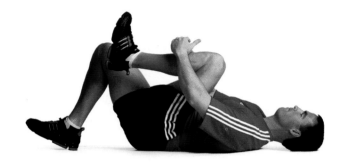

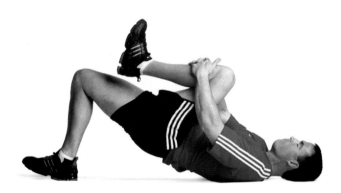

PREHAB

WWW.COREPERFORMANCE.COM

MINI BAND STANDING

PROCEDURE:

Stand with your feet just outside of your hips and a mini band above your knees. Take a partial squat. Keeping your left leg stationary, rotate your right knee in and out for the prescribed number of reps. Then switch legs and repeat.

COACHING KEY:

Keep both feet flat on the ground and your pelvis stable. Don't let the knee of your stationary leg drop in.

YOU SHOULD FEEL IT:

In your glutes.

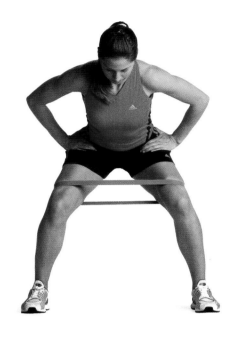

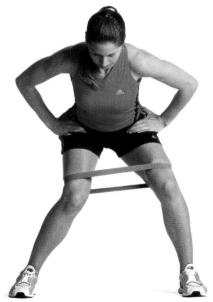

PREHAB

MINI BAND WALKING

PROCEDURE:

Move to the right, pushing with your left leg while stepping laterally with your right leg. Bring your left foot back to the starting position and continue until you've completed your reps on that side. Be sure to keep your knees pushed apart throughout the movement. Repeat while moving to the left.

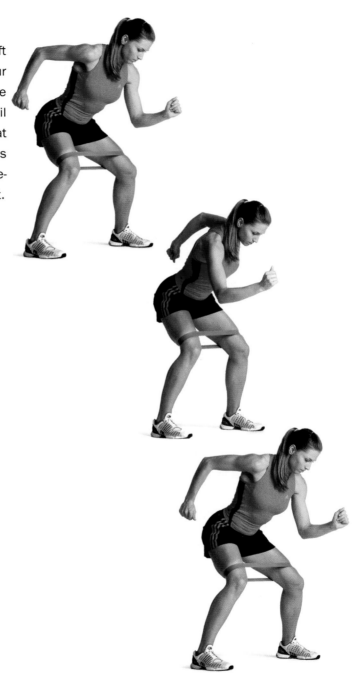

PREHAB

MINI BAND WALKING (ADD RESISTANCE)

PROCEDURE:

Increase the resistance by using a band with greater tension.

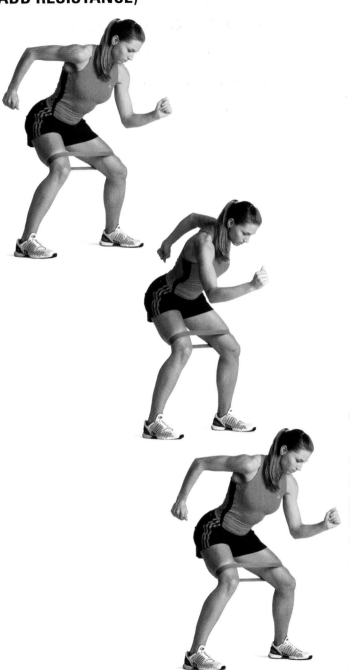

PREHAB

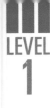

FLOOR *Y*s AND *T*s

PROCEDURE:

Lying facedown on the floor with your arms raised slightly above shoulder height, create a *Y*, with your torso and thumbs up. Glide your shoulder blades toward your spine and lift your arms off the ground. Return to the starting position and repeat to complete your reps. For the *T*, pull your shoulder blades in toward your spine and extend your arms to the sides to create a *T* with your torso.

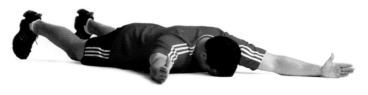

COACHING KEY:

Keep your stomach tight and your thumbs up. Move from the scapulae (the shoulder blades), not from your arms, extending your shoulders and hands.

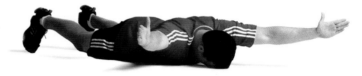

YOU SHOULD FEEL IT:

In your shoulders and upper back.

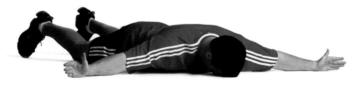

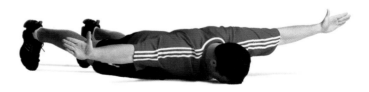

PHYSIOBALL *Y*s AND *T*s (ARMS BENT)

PROCEDURE:

Perform the same exercises with bent elbows on a physioball, lying facedown over the top of the ball so that your back is flat and your chest is off the ball.

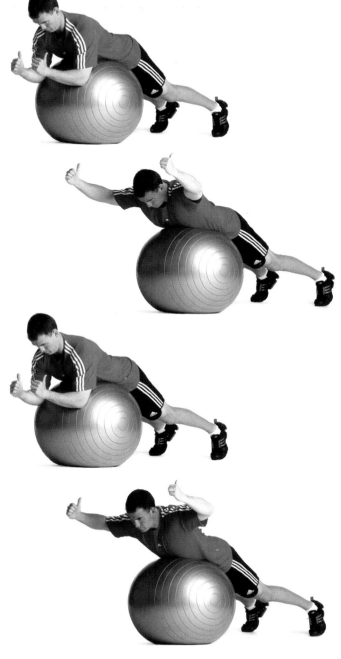

LEVEL 2

PREHAB

PHYSIOBALL *Y*S AND *T*S (ARMS EXTENDED)

PROCEDURE:

Perform the same exercise as for Level 2, but with your arms extended instead of bent.

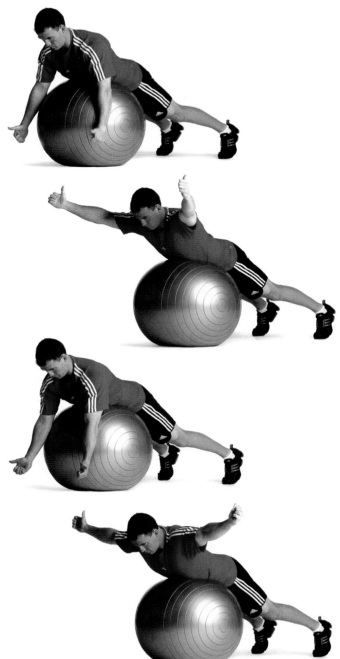

PHYSIOBALL *Y*S AND *T*S (WITH WEIGHT)

PROCEDURE:

Add a light weight—1 to 3 pounds.

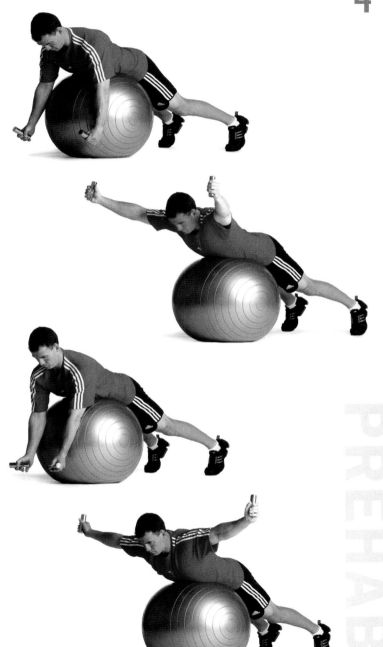

PREHAB

SUMO SQUAT TO HAMSTRING STRETCH

PROCEDURE:

Standing with your feet shoulder width apart, bend at the waist and grab your toes. Drop your hips to the ground, lift your chest up, and then pull your hips forward until your torso is vertical. Maintaining a flat back, push your hips up and back until you feel a stretch in your hamstrings. Drop your hips back to the ground and repeat until you've completed all your reps.

COACHING KEY:

Keep your chest up, your back flat, and your heels on the floor. Keep your elbows inside of your knees. For an easier move, place a $\frac{1}{4}$- to 2-inch block under your heels. As your mobility and stability improve, perform the movement with a smaller and smaller heel lift.

YOU SHOULD FEEL:

A stretch in your hamstrings, groin, lower back, and quads.

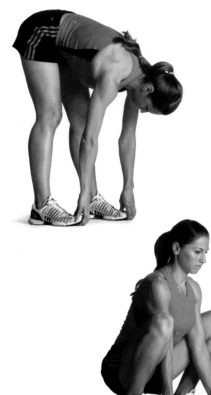

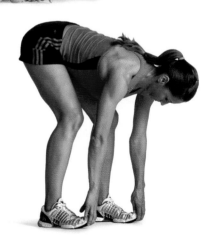

PHYSIOBALL PLATE CRUNCH

PROCEDURE:

Lying on top of the ball, arch your torso over the ball. Try to touch your shoulder blades, back, and glutes over the ball so that your abdominals are completely stretched. Hold the weight plate behind your head. Roll your hips and chest up at the same time while pulling your belly button in. Crunch from the top of your torso and then lower your hips and chest to the starting position.

COACHING KEY:

Arch your torso completely.

YOU SHOULD FEEL:

A stretch in your abs and core.

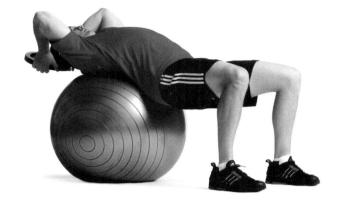

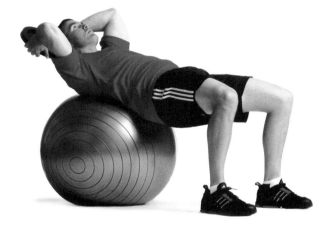

PUSHUP (KNEELING), OR PUSHUP

PROCEDURE:

Assume a pushup position with your hands and knees on the ground. Lower your body to the ground, then reverse the movement without touching the ground. Keep your body in a straight line. If you don't need to kneel, assume the normal pushup position.

COACHING KEY:

Push your sternum as far away from your hands as possible at the end of the movement.

YOU SHOULD FEEL IT:

In your chest, arms, and torso.

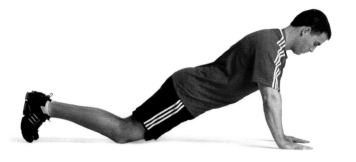

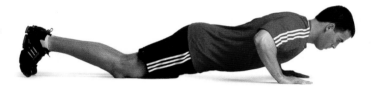

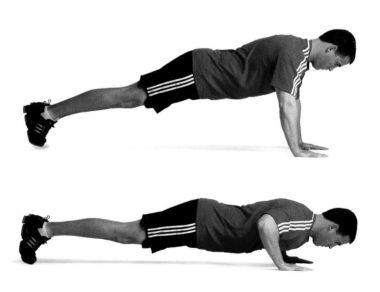

PUSHUP (WITH PHYSIOBALL)

PROCEDURE:

Assume a pushup position, but with your hands on a physioball and your feet on the floor. With your belly button drawn in, lower yourself to the point where your chest barely grazes the ball. Control the ball as you push back up, holding your belly button in and pushing your sternum as far away from the ball as possible. Your shoulder blades should be pushed away from each other in a "plus" position (as far forward as possible) at the top of the movement. Keep your fingers pointed down the sides of the ball.

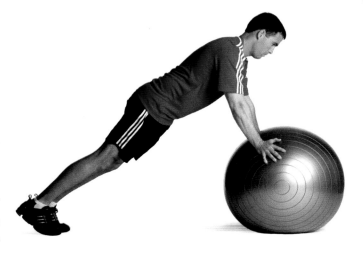

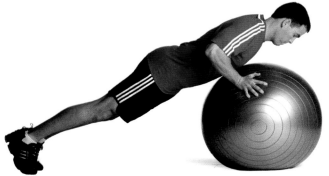

STRENGTH

CORE MOVEMENTS

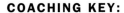

STRENGTH

GLUTE BRIDGE (WITH PHYSIOBALL)

PROCEDURE:

Lie faceup on the ground with your tummy tight and your feet on the ball (or on a bench or a couch). Your legs should be straight, your toes pulled up toward your shins, and your shoulder blades pulled back and down. Contract your glutes to raise your hips until you create a straight line between your ankle and shoulders, so that only your head, shoulders, and arms are touching the floor. Hold for 2 to 3 seconds and repeat until you've completed your reps.

COACHING KEY:

Initiate the movement by firing your glutes, and keep them contracted at the top of the movement. If it is too difficult to balance, spread your arms out to the side. Or, to make it more difficult, cross your arms on your chest.

YOU SHOULD FEEL IT:

In your glutes, hamstrings, and lower back.

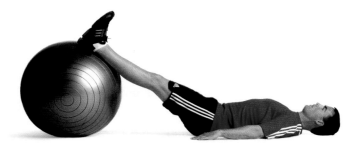

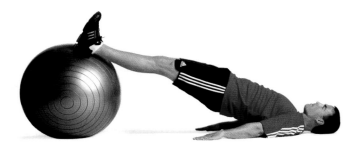

GLUTE BRIDGE (WITH PHYSIOBALL LEG CURL)

PROCEDURE:

Contract your glutes to raise your hips, then pull your heels toward your body. Do not let your hips drop as the ball comes toward you. Extend your legs, then repeat the leg curl for the prescribed number of reps without letting your hips touch the ground.

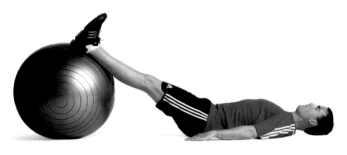

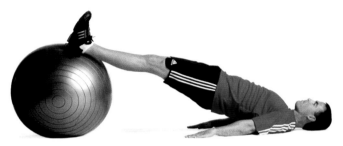

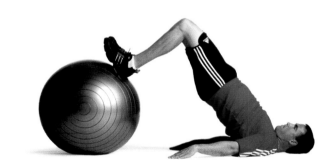

STRENGTH

CORE MOVEMENTS

165

FLOOR CRUNCH

PROCEDURE:

Lie faceup with your knees bent, with a small pad or towel under your lower back to help stretch your abs, and your hands behind your head supporting your neck. Lift your chest until your shoulder blades are off the ground, and at the same time rotate your pelvis toward your belly button. Slowly return to the starting position. Repeat until you've completed your reps.

COACHING KEY:

Do not pull on your head with your hands. Feel each segment of your spine flexing as you crunch and as you stretch over the pad.

YOU SHOULD FEEL IT:

In your abdominals.

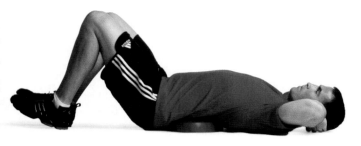

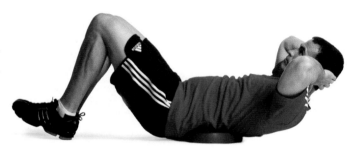

STRENGTH

PHYSIOBALL CRUNCH

PROCEDURE:

Lie faceup with your body arched over the ball and your hands interlocked, supporting your head. Drape your body over the ball—you should feel a mild stretch in your abs. Curl your trunk and pelvis together while keeping your belly button pulled in. Return to the starting position and repeat until you've completed all your reps.

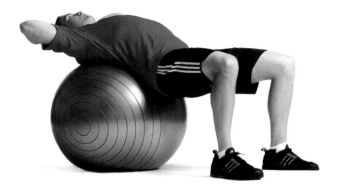

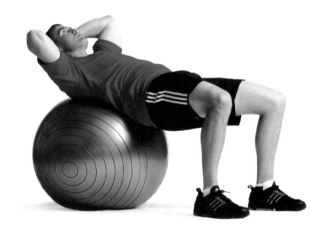

STRENGTH

SQUAT (BODY WEIGHT, WITH MINI BAND)

PROCEDURE:

Stand with your arms at your sides, your feet shoulder width apart and pointing straight ahead, and a mini band around and above your knees. Maintain perfect posture and initiate movement with your hips. As you reach your arms far forward, squat your hips back and down until your thighs are parallel to the floor. Return to a standing position by pushing through your hips. Keep your knees out. Repeat until you've completed all your reps.

COACHING KEY:

Keep your knees behind your toes during the movement. Also, keep your knees pushing out against the band so that they do not collapse to the inside during the movement. If you extend your arms in front of you, you can sit back more comfortably. Keep your chest up and your back flat.

YOU SHOULD FEEL IT:

In your glutes, hamstrings, and quads.

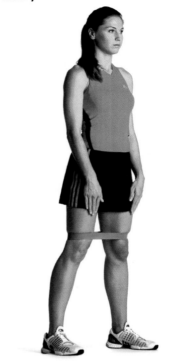

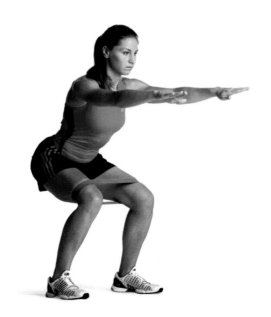

SQUAT (SINGLE LEG)

PROCEDURE:

Stand on one foot in front of a bench or chair, holding 2½- to 5-pound weights in each hand. Initiate movement with your hips, squatting back and down on one leg as you reach forward until your glutes touch the bench. Return to a standing position using only the leg you are balancing on. Repeat for the prescribed number of repetitions, then switch legs. Do not let your knee collapse to the inside.

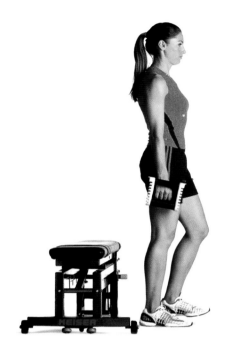

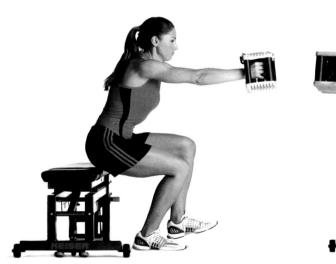

STRENGTH

STRENGTH

SPLIT SQUAT

PROCEDURE:

Hold dumbbells at arm's length at your sides. Place your back foot on a box or bench and step out into a lunge. Lower your hips toward the floor by squatting back and down. Without letting your back knee touch the ground, return to the starting position by driving your weight back up with your front leg. Do all the reps with that leg forward, then switch legs and repeat.

COACHING KEY:

Don't let your front knee slide forward over your toes; if it does, start over again with your front foot farther forward.

YOU SHOULD FEEL IT:

In your hips and the fronts of your legs.

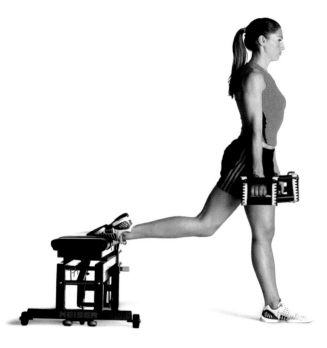

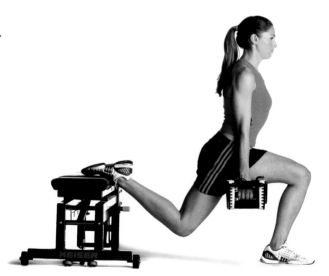

SPLIT DUMBBELL CURL

PROCEDURE:

In a standing position, hold dumbbells at your side and place one leg on a stable object at about midthigh height. Shift your weight forward onto your front leg, taking your back leg into a stretch. Now, keeping your elbows still, lift the dumbbells to your shoulders as you rotate your palms to the ceiling. Return to the starting position and repeat until you've completed all your reps. Switch legs midway through the set.

COACHING KEY:

Keep your stomach and the glute muscles of your rear leg tight throughout the movement. Do not allow your back to move. Do not rock forward or backward, and don't move your elbows.

YOU SHOULD FEEL IT:

In your biceps, glutes, and hip flexors.

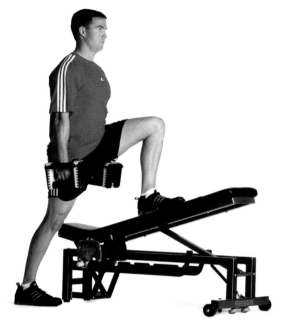

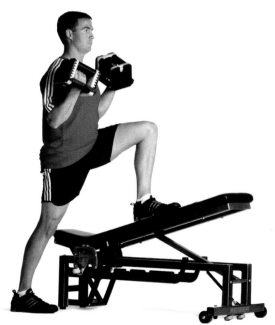

STRENGTH

SPLIT DUMBBELL CURL TO PRESS

PROCEDURE:

After performing a biceps curl, press the weight over your head, finishing with your palms facing forward. Switch legs midway through the set.

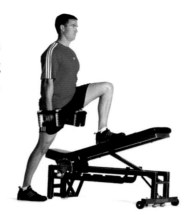

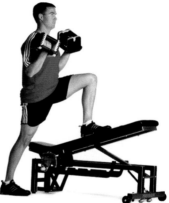

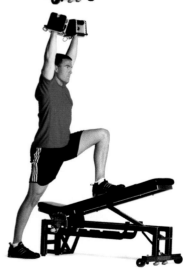

WWW.COREPERFORMANCE.COM

ALTERNATING SPLIT DUMBBELL CURL TO PRESS

PROCEDURE:

Stand holding dumbbells at your sides with your front foot resting on a bench or sturdy step at about midthigh height. Push your body weight slightly forward, with your back glute tight. Perform a biceps curl so that the dumbbells are at your chest. Press your right hand over your head as you lower the left. As you lower your right hand, repeat the motion with your left arm so that the dumbbells pass at your torso. Repeat for the prescribed number of repetitions, switching the foot on the bench halfway through the set. Contract the glute of your back leg to stabilize yourself. Switch legs midway through the set.

COACHING KEY:

Maintain perfect posture, with your belly button pulled in and your shoulder blades pulled back and down. Do not let your back arch when the weight is pressed overhead.

YOU SHOULD FEEL IT:

In your biceps and shoulders, and throughout your pillar.

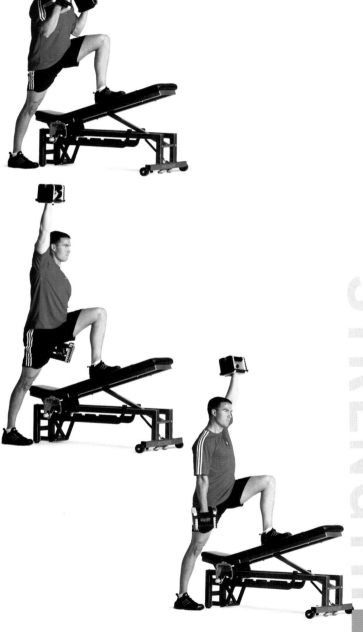

STRENGTH

STANDING LIFT

PROCEDURE:

Squat, rotating from left to right while holding a weight plate. Square up and press the plate over your head.

COACHING KEY:

Keep your chest up and your back flat. This exercise combines the familiar movements of squatting, rotating, the upright row, and the incline press. Lower in the same pattern as you lifted.

YOU SHOULD FEEL IT:

In your hips, torso rotators, upper back, chest, and shoulders.

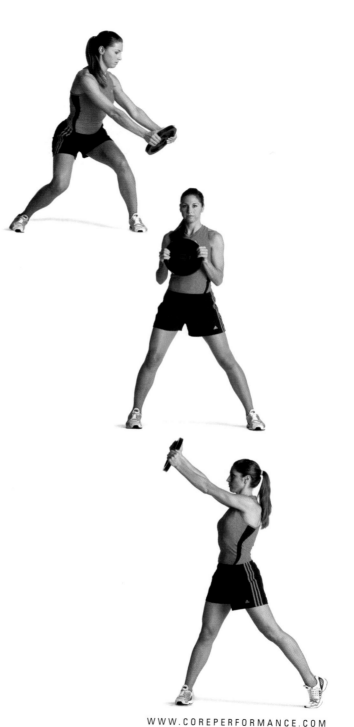

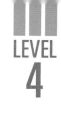

STANDING LIFT (ONE LEG)

PROCEDURE:

Stand holding a weight plate or dumbbell in a low position, or holding a rope handle attached to a low pulley cable. Your foot should be perpendicular to the cable if you are using one, your hips should be flexed, and your abdominals should be drawn in. Balance on your inside foot, turn your shoulders and hip toward the leg that's supporting your weight, and keep your chest up and your stomach tight. Squat down so that the weight is outside this leg, then fire from your glutes and torso. Pull the weight or handles toward your chest while extending your supporting leg. Turn your trunk away from your supporting leg as your hands push up and away. Return to the starting position and repeat to complete your reps, then switch legs.

COACHING KEY:

Keep your chest up and your back flat. Your torso will rotate from start to finish. This exercise combines the familiar movements of balance squatting, rotating, the upright row, and the incline press. Lower in the same pattern as you lifted.

YOU SHOULD FEEL IT:

In your hips, torso rotators, upper back, chest, and shoulders.

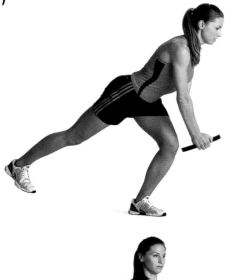

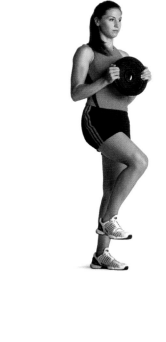

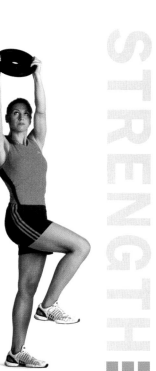

STRENGTH

STRENGTH

ALTERNATING DUMBBELL BENCH PRESS

PROCEDURE:

Lie faceup on a bench, holding dumb-bells at the outside edges of your shoulders, your palms facing your thighs. Lift the dumbbells straight up over your chest. Keeping one arm straight, lower the other dumbbell, touch the outside of your shoulder, then push it back up. Switch arms and continue to alternate arms for the pre-scribed number of repetitions.

COACHING KEY:

Keep your nonworking arm straight. Keep your feet on the floor and your hips and shoulders on the bench at all times. Pull your stomach in to stabilize your core.

YOU SHOULD FEEL IT:

In your chest, shoulders, and triceps.

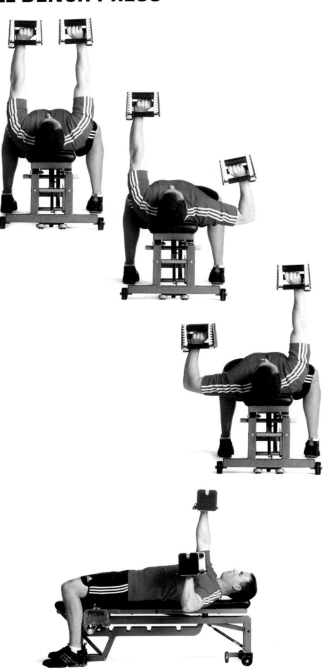

176

ROMANIAN DEADLIFT (TWO ARMS, ONE LEG)

PROCEDURE:

Stand on one foot while holding a dumbbell in each hand, using an overhand grip. "Hinge" over at the waist, lowering the dumbbells as your non-supporting leg lifts behind you. Return to the standing position by contracting your hamstrings and glutes. Repeat for the prescribed number of repetitions, then switch legs.

COACHING KEY:

Do not let your back arch. Your torso and leg should move as one unit. Fire the glute of your extended leg to keep it straight. Keep your shoulder blades back and down throughout the movement, and keep the dumbbells close to your shin.

YOU SHOULD FEEL IT:

In your glutes, hamstrings, and back.

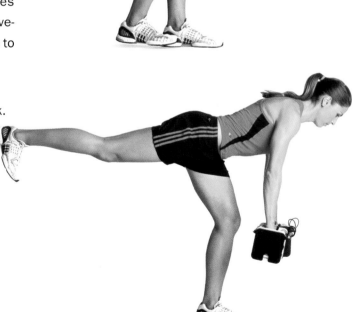

STRENGTH

ONE-ARM, ONE-LEG DUMBBELL ROW

PROCEDURE:

Stand on your right leg, hinged over at the waist, holding a dumbbell with your right hand and holding on to a stable, waist-high surface with your left hand. Lift your left leg to form a *T* with your body. Slide your right shoulder blade toward your spine and then lift the weight to your body by driving your elbow to the ceiling. Return to the starting position and repeat for the prescribed number of repetitions. Then switch sides.

COACHING KEY:

Move with your shoulder, not your arm, to initiate the row. Keep your back level—your shoulders should stay parallel to the floor—and fire the glute of your extended leg to keep it parallel to the floor. Extend the leg opposite the hand doing the lifting.

YOU SHOULD FEEL IT:

In your back, lats, and shoulders.

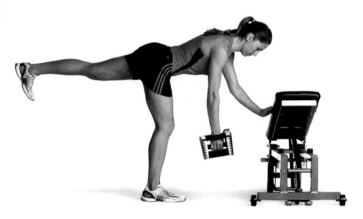

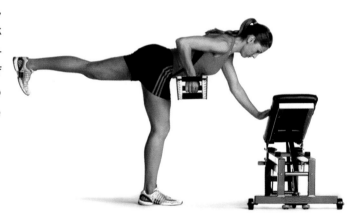

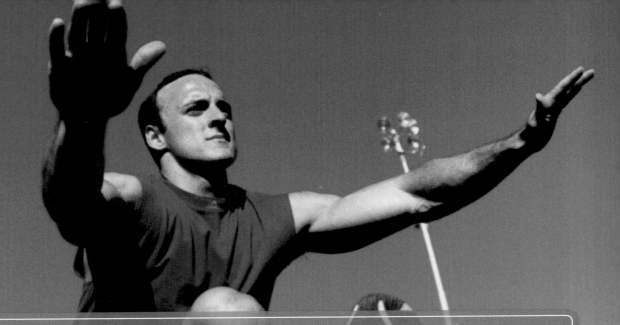 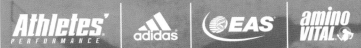   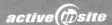

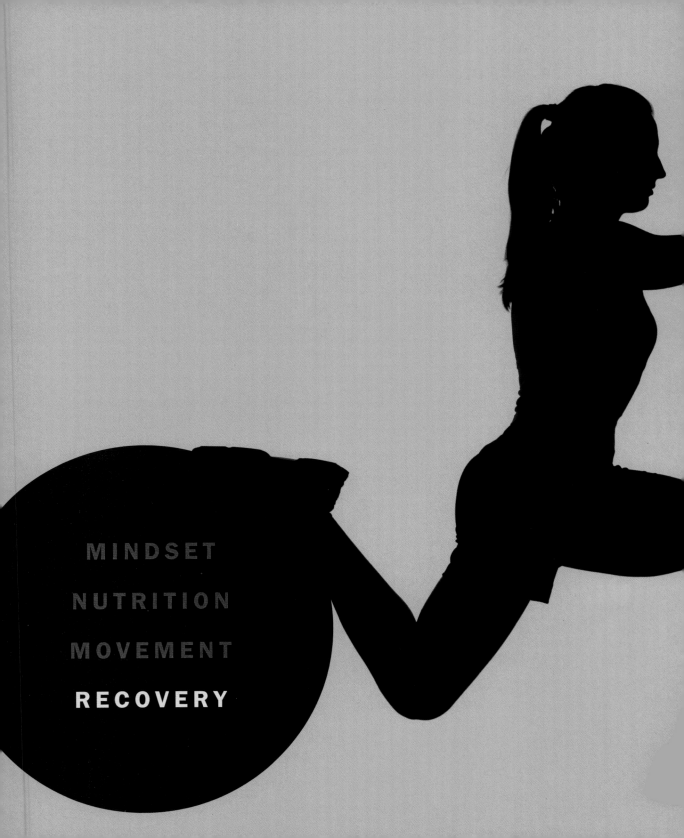

MINDSET

NUTRITION

MOVEMENT

RECOVERY

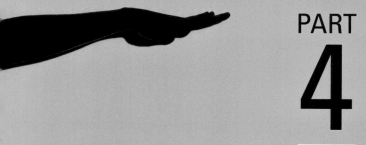

CORE
RECOVERY
AND
INTEGRATION

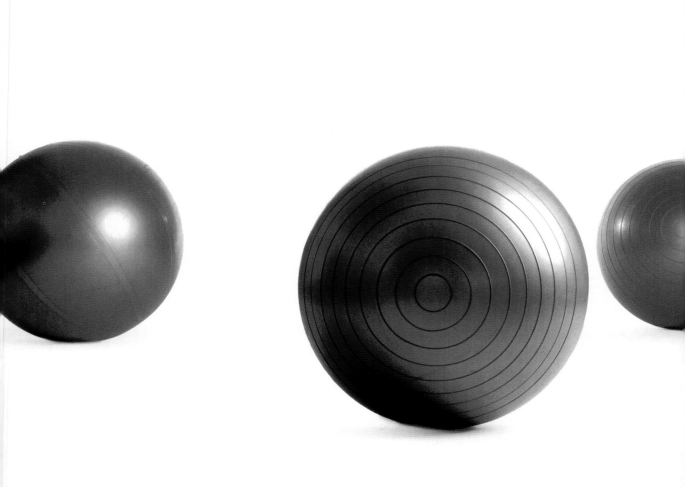

REGENERATION

W hether it's working out or simply working at the office, it's impossible to go all-out, all the time. You need some time to recover, a process I call regeneration.

Regeneration is a lifestyle philosophy, a recognition that you need to plan ways to recover—mentally and physically—in all areas of your life. You actually experience the benefit of your hard work on the days that you rest and repair your body.

There's a big difference between rest—doing nothing at all—and "active rest." In this program, you work hard on Mondays, Wednesdays, and Fridays, and devote Tuesdays and Thursdays to cardio work. If that's all that your schedule permits, fine—this program was designed for the working person. It no doubt will take some effort to carve out time to work out on weekdays, and more likely than not, you won't have the time or inclination to exercise on the weekends.

I can appreciate that, and I applaud you for your efforts. But as you become more proficient with this program, you might be looking for more. You could take some combination of Tuesday, Thursday, Saturday, and Sunday and take a break from serious training but still do things that benefit your body, such as

WORK + REST = SUCCESS

Do you actively work recovery into your daily schedule? Into your yearly schedule?

Do you actively work recovery into your weekly exercise plan?

Do you understand the effective methods to recover, and do you allow your body to constantly regenerate to meet the demands of life?

playing golf, tennis, or basketball. You're not training per se, but you're still getting the benefit of physical activity. Not only that, you're having fun.

Regeneration is crucial for the body to experience the gains it made by working out. It's why we're not going to train superhard every day, and it's why we'll take 48-hour breaks before revisiting elements of the Core Workout.

First, ask yourself the three questions above in "Work + Rest = Success."

"Regen" is not just a physical philosophy. The time spent at rest is when we enjoy the fruits of our labor. Not only that, but we also recharge our batteries and come back invigorated and stronger, ready to perform at even higher levels.

If you're working hard all the time, you're never truly recovered. You might be working hard, but you're not working smart. On the contrary—you're so mentally and physically fatigued that you're not nearly as productive as you think you are.

Remember, this program will only be moderately successful if you have a limiting lifestyle, and for many people that limitation comes in the form of a lack of sleep. Sleep is a vital component of regeneration.

I see this even with elite athletes, especially younger ones. They have boundless energy and live nocturnal lifestyles, partying into the wee hours and getting little sleep. But even if they don't drink excessively, a couple of beers or cocktails inhibit sleep and contribute to weight gain.

While on the topic of alcohol, remember that earlier we discussed the health benefits of *moderate* consumption of red wine. But remember also that it's difficult to reap the rewards of this program if recreational drinking is a key part of your lifestyle. (It goes without saying that smoking is counterproductive to healthy living.)

Sleep, though, is the most underrated aspect of a healthy lifestyle. Recent studies suggest that the less sleep you get, the more likely you are to be obese. Sleep deprivation

"The ability to do the things I've always wanted to do"

NAME: SOREN ORLEY

AGE: 49

HOMETOWN: ANCHORAGE, ALASKA

Soren Orley had always maintained an active lifestyle. An avid cross-country skier who spends many weekends working for the Alaska Mountain Rescue Group, he prided himself on fitness, even though he had packed on some extra weight in his forties.

In June 2004, for his 48th birthday, his wife gave him a bicycle. He began riding frequently, only to put on a mysterious 12 pounds in less than a week. Though he felt queasy and short of breath, he chalked it up to being allergic to cats.

Doctors diagnosed him with an enlarged heart and pulmonary hypertension, likely a congenital defect. His body was retaining fluid. Two weeks later, Orley underwent surgery to repair an aortic valve.

While undergoing the hospital's rehabilitation program and waiting 7 weeks for clearance to begin strenuous physical activity, Orley read *Core Performance*. He figured it was the right program for him, especially after watching more advanced rehabilitation patients go through "what seemed like a pretty wimpy program."

The medical staff gave him clearance, and within 3 months, his weight dropped to 192, down from a high of 241 before the surgery. He bought pants with a 34-inch waist—4 inches narrower than before. But the more telling results came in flexibility and balance, especially while skiing.

"Before, if a ski caught something, it usually meant an instant face-plant in the snow," says Sorley, a CPA in charge of budget and finance for the University of Alaska–Anchorage. "Now I'm able to adjust and keep going. It's the little things that you notice most about the program."

Orley is back on duty with the Alaska Mountain Rescue Group, which sometimes requires hiking long distances with a 65-pound pack strapped to his back. "When you're hanging off the side of a mountain in a blizzard, trying to keep people alive, you need all of the strength, balance, and flexibility you can muster."

Orley's biggest reward came in the summer of 2005, when one of his daughters graduated from high school and he joined her on a "sea-to-summit-to-sea tour." They biked 200 miles from Ocean Shores, Washington, to Rainier National Park, where they climbed Mt. Rainier and then made the 200-mile return trip.

Not bad for a guy less than a year removed from major open-heart surgery.

"It's not just about how much weight you can lift or how many pounds you lose," Orley says. "Those things are meaningful, but more important, this program has given me the ability to do the things I've always wanted to do."

decreases levels of a hormone called leptin that makes you feel full, and it increases levels of a hunger hormone called ghrelin. It's yet another vicious cycle: Less sleep makes you fat, and being fat impedes your sleep. The National Sleep Foundation estimates that 63 percent of American adults don't get the recommended 8 hours of sleep a night. Also according to the National Sleep Foundation, sleep deprivation and sleep disorders cost Americans more than $100 billion annually in lost productivity, sick leave, and medical expenses.

For all the talk of improving diet and exercise, we tend to ignore this obvious lifestyle component. Throughout this program, I want you to make the best use of your time and get the most benefit, whether it's working out, eating, or even sleeping. You probably know to get 8 hours of sleep a night. But you might not know that it's possible to improve the quality of your sleep by thinking in terms of 90-minute cycles.

The longer you're asleep, the longer you experience rapid-eye-movement (REM) sleep, a period marked by increased brain activity and muscle relaxation. Sleep cycles last approximately 90 minutes, and at the end of each cycle, you start to come out of sleep. Like the groundhog that rises up to look for his shadow, your body senses whether or not it can go into another sleep cycle.

If you're awakened in the middle of a sleep cycle by an alarm clock or a dream, you tend to be disoriented and end up feeling sluggish for much of the day. But if you can manage to wake up at the top of a 90-minute cycle, perhaps with the use of an alarm clock, you'll feel more alert and invigorated.

Sleeping 6 hours might feel more restful than 7 hours if you get up at the top of a sleep cycle. Ideally, you should aim for $7\frac{1}{2}$ to 8 hours, but since many people struggle to get 6 hours of sleep, let's recognize that 6 hours of sleep can be a good thing—provided it's 6 hours of quality sleep, not sleep affected by alcohol—or by sugary foods eaten not long before bedtime.

On the following pages, we've provided some effective regeneration-oriented exercises to use with the rest of the Core Workout routines. By using two simple items—a foam roll and a stretch rope—you can achieve some tremendous results. The foam roll is like a massage. It uses deep compression to help roll out the muscle spasms that develop over time. The rope routine is especially helpful with flexibility. You need not think of the foam roll and rope routine as additional work; just use them while watching TV or at the end of the day before going to bed.

Apply a pattern of rest and regeneration to balance all aspects of your life on a daily, weekly, and yearly basis, and you'll be amazed at how high the quality of your life becomes.

Chapter 11 Summary: Regeneration is a recognition that you need to plan ways to recover in all areas of your life. That way, you'll experience the benefit of work on the days you rest. (Remember: Work + Rest = Success.)

The time spent at rest is when we clear our minds and enjoy the fruits of our labor, when we realize the gains produced by all of our hard work. Not only that, we also recharge our batteries and come back invigorated and stronger, ready to perform at even higher levels. Sleep is a vital component of regeneration. And proper nutrition helps the body regenerate effectively.

SELF-MASSAGE ROUTINE

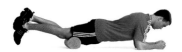

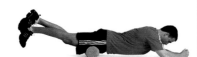

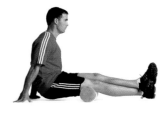

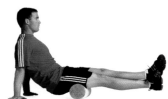

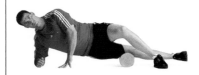

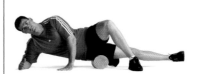

FOAM ROLL QUADRICEPS/HIP FLEXOR

Lie facedown on the floor with a foam roll under the front of your thighs. Roll over the quads from your hip to just above your knee. For added benefit, cross one leg over the other, placing all your body weight on the front of one thigh. The more uncomfortable it feels, the more that muscle needs to be massaged. Hold your position on sore spots for an extended time to release the soreness. Roll slightly on the outside and inside of the thighs as well as down the front of the thighs, as if you were getting a massage.

FOAM ROLL HAMSTRING

Sit on the floor and place a foam roll under the back of one thigh with your other leg crossed. Roll over the foam, moving it up and down the length of the back of your thigh. If it is too sensitive, uncross your legs and roll both hamstrings at once. The more uncomfortable it is, the more that muscle needs to be massaged. Hold your position on sore spots for an extended time to release the soreness, as if you were getting a massage.

FOAM ROLL IT BAND

Lie on your side with a foam roll under the outside of your thigh. Roll over the foam from your hip to just above your knee. The more uncomfortable it is, the more that muscle needs to be massaged. Hold your position on sore spots for an extended time to release soreness, as if you were getting a massage.

REGENERATION

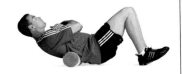

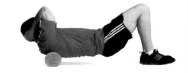

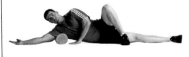

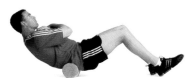

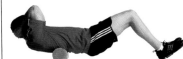

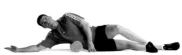

FOAM ROLL LOWER BACK

Lie faceup with a foam roll under your midback. Cross your arms over your chest. Roll from the middle of your back down to the base of your spine and repeat. The more uncomfortable it is, the more that muscle needs to be massaged. Hold your position on sore spots for an extended time to release the soreness, as if you were getting a massage.

FOAM ROLL UPPER BACK

Lie faceup with a foam roll under your upper back. Hold your hands behind your head with your elbows pointed to the sky. Roll from your shoulders down to the middle of your back and repeat. The more uncomfortable it is, the more that muscle needs to be massaged. Hold your position on sore spots for an extended time to release the soreness, as if you were getting a massage.

FOAM ROLL LATS

Lie on your side with a foam roll under your armpit. Roll from the side of your lower back up to your armpit. The more uncomfortable it is, the more that muscle needs to be massaged. Hold your position on sore spots for an extended time to release the soreness, as if you were getting a massage.

FLEXIBILITY ROUTINE

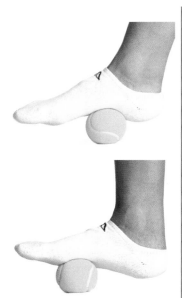

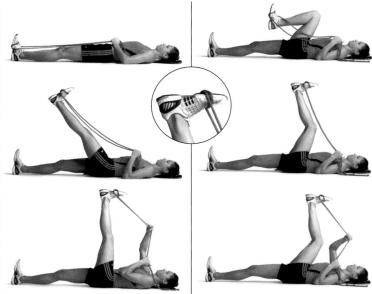

ARCH ROLL (TENNIS BALL)

Standing with your shoes off, place one foot on a tennis ball. Roll the arch of your foot back and forth over the tennis ball. The more uncomfortable it is, the more that muscle needs to be massaged. Hold your position on sore spots for an extended time to release the soreness. Roll through different angles to cover entire arch completely, as if you were getting a deep massage.

ROPE STRETCH— STRAIGHT LEG HAMSTRING

Lie on your back with your left leg straight and a rope wrapped around your foot. Actively lift your left leg as far as possible, pulling the rope above your head, then give it gentle assistance with the rope until a stretch is felt. Hold for 2 seconds and then relax. Repeat. Keep the opposite leg on the floor by pushing your heel as far away from your head as possible, contracting the glute. You should feel a stretch in the hamstring of your raised leg and a stretch in the hip flexor of your bottom leg.

ROPE STRETCH— BENT-KNEE HAMSTRING

Lie on your back with your left knee pulled to your chest and a rope wrapped around your foot. Actively straighten your left knee as much as possible without letting it move away from your chest, pulling the rope above your head. It is okay if the knee is not able to straighten fully. Give it gentle assistance with the rope until a stretch is felt, hold for 2 seconds, and then relax. Repeat for the prescribed number of repetitions.

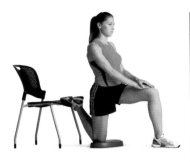

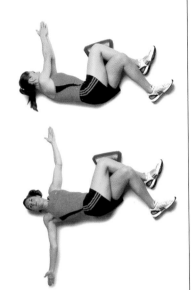

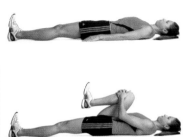

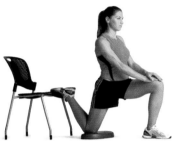

QUAD/HIP FLEXOR STRETCH (KNEELING, BACK FOOT UP)

Place your back knee on a soft mat or pad with your back foot elevated on a chair or a physioball. While keeping a slight forward lean of the torso, tighten the core and the glute of the leg with the knee on the ground. Maintaining this posture, shift your entire body slightly forward. Exhale and hold the stretch for 2 seconds. Relax and repeat. Avoid excessive arching in your back. You should feel a stretch in the front of your hip and your upper thigh.

90/90 STRETCH

Lie faceup on the floor with your arms out to the side, your left knee bent to 90 degrees, and your right leg crossed over the left. Roll over onto your left side, pinning a pad between your right knee and the ground. While maintaining pressure on the pad and keeping your hips still, rotate your chest and right arm back to the right, trying to put your back on the ground. Hold for 2 seconds and then return to the starting position. Repeat for the prescribed number of repetitions and then switch sides.

GLUTE STRETCH (SUPINE)

Lying faceup on ground, actively lift one knee to your chest and then give it gentle assistance by grabbing the knee and pulling it closer to your chest. Exhale and hold the stretch for 2 seconds, then return to the starting position. Repeat for the prescribed number of repetitions and switch legs. Keep your nonstretching leg flat on the floor by pushing the bottom of your heel away from your head. You should feel a stretch in your glutes, hamstrings, and hip flexors.

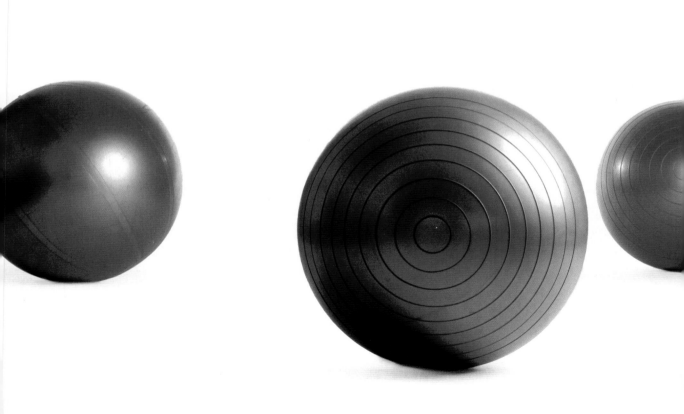

QUALITY OF TIME

I f you've ever watched an hourglass, you've witnessed an optical illusion. At first, the sand seems to pass through the narrow opening slowly. But the more sand passes through, the faster it seems to progress.

The same is true with time. The older we get, the more quickly time appears to pass. We know that this is not *literally* true, but the fast-paced adult life seems to fly by more quickly than what we remember as children, when the last hour of the school day or the final weeks before the winter holidays seemed to go on forever.

Time is the limiting factor for everyone and the biggest obstacle to leading a healthy lifestyle. After all, everyone wants to exercise, but they can't find the time. Everyone wants to eat healthier meals, but they only have time to grab something quick. Everyone wants to get more sleep and rely less on caffeine, but who has the time?

Now that we've addressed these challenges, we need to look at time from a broader perspective. We need a framework to execute these new strategies. Everything we do within our Core Essentials sphere will only work if it's an integrated lifestyle.

Most of us purchase day planners and desk calendars in December, mapping out all of the important events for the following year. These days, it's possible to do it all electronically.

In theory, this exercise is supposed to provide structure and organization to our lives, and to some degree it does. But it also causes us to look short-term, at the upcoming day or week, and be reactive, like a goalie.

Instead, why don't we map out the year on one sheet of paper? (See the planning calendars provided on pages 198 and 199.) You can still use your daily or weekly planners, but it will be easier to concentrate on the most important things and find chunks of time where you can make a difference.

You have Monday through Sunday at a glance. This will help you be more proactive. Take a highlighter and block out the week between Christmas and New Year's, Thanksgiving week, and any weeklong vacations in the school calendar if you have children or are a student yourself.

When you do this, it not only makes things seem more manageable, but it enables you to see smaller 6-week and 8-week windows where you can set up process-oriented goals. For instance, for the first 6-week block, we already have set realistic goals of working out three times a week, along with purging your pantry of unhealthy foods and stocking it with better choices.

Break this up into chunks, adapting it to your lifestyle. Otherwise, it might seem overwhelming. You might figure, "Wow, I've got this trip coming up in March, and then the kids are out for a week in April, and we're traveling over the holidays this year. There's just no way."

If you break up the time, your plan doesn't seem so ambitious. It also speaks to the key component of recovery. You can't work out diligently or go to the office 7 days a week, every week. Your body and soul would not allow it. You have to know that there's some built-in reward in the form of weekends and vacation. That time allows you to recharge and come back even stronger.

Think of how hard you work before vacation. You scramble to make sure everything is done at the office and that someone covers for you in the event that something comes up in your absence. At home, you put the house in order, arrange for pet care, and stop the mail and newspapers. You move at a furious pace because of that dangling carrot of vacation.

The same is true with this program. If you know there's a break in the workout routine or a break in your schedule, in the form of vacation, it will inspire you to work that much more efficiently.

No matter how we structure our lives, we have to work hard. Vince Lombardi, the legendary football coach of the Green Bay Packers, famously remarked that "the only place success comes before work is in the dictionary."

No matter how proactive we are in terms of scheduling and structuring our lives, there will be things we can't control. There's a part of every day where you just have to stand up

"I'm outdriving the guys!"

NAME: JANET OJA

AGE: 44

HOMETOWN: KAYSVILLE, UTAH

Janet Oja always considered herself a pretty good athlete. The Core program alleviated some recurring shoulder problems, but the biggest benefit she received was finding the confidence to try sports that require not only core strength but also mental toughness.

These days, she enjoys "canyoneering," exploring the canyons near her Utah home through a combination of hiking, swimming, rappelling, and rock climbing.

"I had always wanted to try rock climbing, but, like a lot of women, I didn't think that I had the upper body strength," she says. "Now I know that anyone can generate this tremendous core strength."

Not long after starting the program, she began to outpace her husband on bicycle rides. She noticed while hiking that her balance was significantly better. Climbing hills was much easier. The most telling sign came when she started outdriving her male counterparts on the golf course.

"I always thought I was centered and balanced on the golf course, but now I'm not falling off the back of my shoes," says Oja, a medical technologist. "I feel the difference constantly, whether I'm picking up a bag of groceries or if I slip while hiking. Now, I automatically catch myself and don't miss a beat.

"It's like rediscovering sports all over again. Every time I participate in a sport, whether I've done it before or not, I always anticipate how the Core program has enhanced how well I 'play.' I am never disappointed."

Oja, who does her core training in the basement of her home, has introduced the program to her two sons, who play football and baseball. Having completed marathons and triathlons, she's hardly lacking in competitive drive, but she says her core training has given her the confidence to attempt anything physical.

"Even in my forties, I can still pick up new things, which is amazing," she says. "This program has allowed me to dream bigger."

to the demands of life, even if that means playing goalie. I run several successful businesses, with employees and clients that require attention, and some days I'm just stopping shots.

The key is to improve our efficiency—our quality of time—and work smarter. A friend of mine once gave me a terrific compliment, saying he was continually amazed by my ability to show a greater capacity for work. At first, I was taken aback. I make it a priority to spend time with family and friends and on things I enjoy. I don't think of myself as a workaholic.

But what my friend meant was that I find a way to get more done in the same period of time; I continually work more efficiently—and it starts with my health. No matter how busy I become, I must get that daily exercise in and eat properly.

So, I schedule that time like any other appointment. In addition to my one-sheet, 365-day calendar, I keep a weekly calendar that includes a weekday workout at 6:15 a.m. I exercise for no more than 60 minutes, and usually just 30, but I'm able to make that workout progressively more efficient and thus more effective, along with an active day.

For many people, the only time to work out will be the first thing in the morning. That sets a good tone for the rest of the day and provides you with a powerful endorphin rush to tackle the tasks ahead. For stay-at-home parents, that's the worst time of day since there are kids who need attention. Perhaps you can schedule your workout around school or naptime. (If that's too unpredictable, a growing number of fitness chains provide the equivalent of 1- or 2-hour daycare right in the gym.)

No matter how busy you are, there is a window of opportunity. Start by looking at the broad, yearlong picture. Set some manageable goals, and then find that one period of the day where you can make it happen, and schedule it. This is no different from what I do with professional athletes. We take their yearlong schedule and daily routines of practice and games and work in training around it.

I know, I know; if you had an exciting, high-paying job contingent on being in top physical condition, you too would feel inspired to work out harder. But here's the funny little secret of my business: Most athletes, because of the grueling travel and rigid schedule of competition and practices, plus family, do not have much time for day-to-day conditioning. The reason they are world class is that they find the time in their day.

That's great for my business since they take advantage of 4- to 6-week visits to my facilities for some intense training. The rest of the year, we support them with programs to maintain their bodies throughout the season.

When you look at your yearlong calendar, you will find periods where it might be impossible to do much. That's okay. The point is to have a program in place where you can do *something*

during those periods and be focused the rest of the time.

The goal, of course, is to have goals, not to just play goaltender. How many times does New Year's Eve roll around and we wonder where the year went and what we have to show for it? It's like the person who has worked in the same position for 15 years. Has his career seen steady progression, or does he just have 1 year of experience repeated 15 times over?

We don't just want to maintain our lives; we want to constantly make them more efficient and productive so that we can enjoy more. It starts with our physical health. Our bodies are the vehicles for our success, and it's a lot easier to stay motivated when you know that it's not just about you. As a centered self, it's about how you can help and elevate others.

Chapter 12 Summary: We want to make the most of our time by looking at the calendar in terms of measurable chunks. Whether finding time to work out or looking to fit in all of our work and personal commitments, we want to find windows of opportunity and set manageable, process-oriented goals. You'll find that within this structure you can accomplish almost anything.

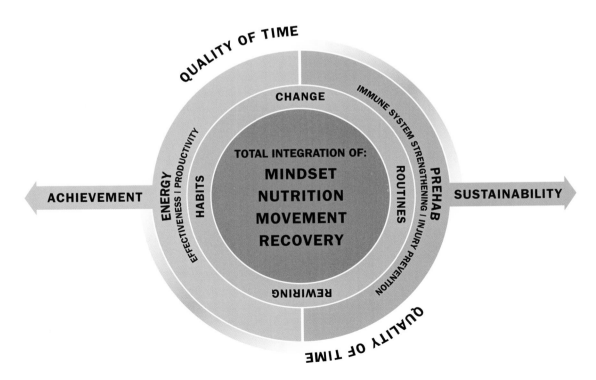

2006 ANNUAL PLANNING CALENDAR

	EVENT	MONDAY	TUESDAY	WEDNESDAY	THURSDAY	FRIDAY	SATURDAY	SUNDAY
JAN	2							
	9							
	16							
	23							
	30							
FEB	6							
	13							
	20							
	27							
MAR	6							
	13							
	20							
	27							
APR	3							
	10							
	17							
	24							
MAY	1							
	8							
	15							
	22							
	29							
JUN	5							
	12							
	19							
	26							
JUL	3							
	10							
	17							
	24							
	31							
AUG	7							
	14							
	21							
	28							
SEP	4							
	11							
	18							
	25							
OCT	2							
	9							
	16							
	23							
	30							
NOV	6							
	13							
	20							
	27							
DEC	4							
	11							
	18							
	25							

2007 ANNUAL PLANNING CALENDAR

EVENT		MONDAY	TUESDAY	WEDNESDAY	THURSDAY	FRIDAY	SATURDAY	SUNDAY
JAN	1							
	8							
	15							
	22							
	29							
FEB	5							
	12							
	19							
	26							
MAR	5							
	12							
	19							
	26							
APR	2							
	9							
	16							
	23							
	30							
MAY	7							
	14							
	21							
	28							
JUN	4							
	11							
	18							
	25							
JUL	2							
	9							
	16							
	23							
	30							
AUG	6							
	13							
	20							
	27							
SEP	3							
	10							
	17							
	24							
OCT	1							
	8							
	15							
	22							
	29							
NOV	5							
	12							
	19							
	26							
DEC	3							
	10							
	17							
	24							
	31							

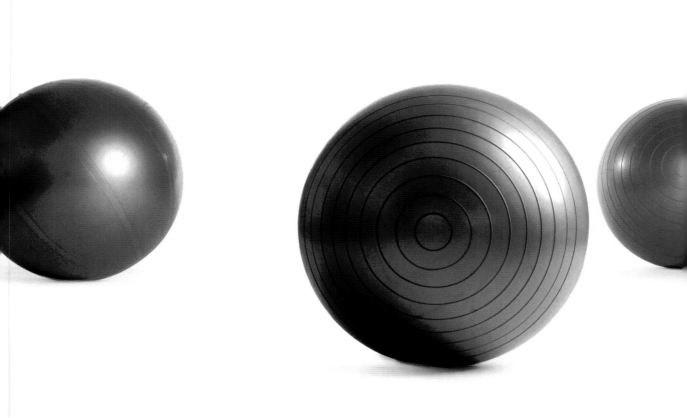

CHAPTER 13

KEEPING SCORE

n my previous book, *Core Performance,* we issued a challenge to readers to send us their feedback about the program. The greatest reward of writing that book was that I got to hear from folks who used the Core system to overcome pain, lose weight, increase flexibility, and install a plan of high-performance nutrition and exercise for long-term health and success.

You've heard from some of those people in this book. We brought others out to our Athletes' Performance training facility in Tempe, Arizona, for a special week of training so they could share with me firsthand how the Core program has impacted their lives.

Thousands of people have joined our online high-performance community at www. coreperformance.com. Each week, we answer their questions about the Core program and provide them with the latest scientific information on nutrition, fitness, and performance. I hope you'll join this growing community of people who have made the commitment to a lifetime of high performance.

This is an ongoing process. You'll notice that we did not put a time frame on this program. There was no "12 Weeks to a Better You" slogan, no "6-Week Plan for Success" subtitle. We presented *Core Performance* as a 12-week plan because, well, that's what everyone in the world of fitness book publishing tends to do. We found that most people wanted more. They didn't wish to repeat the 12-week cycle or the latter stages; they were looking for more progression.

We assembled this program with the goal of using as little equipment as possible. We wanted to eliminate excuses for not working out, while providing an efficient program that will allow you to succeed regardless of your financial resources. By following this program, you will achieve great results.

But perhaps you have a little more money to spend. And, if you do, there are some tools we provide that can help you train even more efficiently to thrive in the Game of Life.

This book's Web site, www.coreperformance. com, is the home for the products and programs we have developed and tested that will complement your Core training program.

First, check out our online Core Store. We have assembled several tools, based on the book, that are great resources for the Core Performance Essentials program, whether you prefer to work out at home or in a gym. I know many of you have told me that you love our workouts, and wish I could be there to lead you through them. Well, along these lines, we have created a Core Performance Essentials DVD series, in which I lead you through the various 30-minute workouts right in your living room.

Alternatively, you'll find in the Core Store a set of laminated cards featuring each level of the workouts with exercise pictures. These cards are a great tool to remind you of proper form as you work out at home or the gym.

Also in the Core Store, we have assembled several packages to create a Core Gym at home. I know that you are incredibly busy, and maybe a gym membership is just not feasible, or maybe you have a membership but are never able to use it for lack of time. A simple Core home gym lets you build the Core program around *your* life.

Maybe you're thinking, "Sure, that would be great, but I don't have the time or space for elaborate equipment." The beauty of this is that the equipment is compact and easy to use.

Our equipment partner, GoFit, has teamed with us to compile several, affordable packages of equipment that you can purchase with a single click in the Core Store. Of course, you also can purchase individual pieces of equipment to fit your needs.

Once you've checked out the Core Store, you will notice a whole world of Core Performance programs available on the Web site. If you're new to the Core Performance community and just getting the hang of taking charge of your body and your life, I want you to focus on this book and mastering the program. We tried to make this book all-encompassing, and indeed, if you just keep trying to pack more and more into your 30-minute workouts, this book might be all you ever need.

But if you're someone who wants to commit a little more time, or if you've caught the Core "bug" and want to take your game to higher levels, check out the programs available.

These programs include the original *Core Performance* book (now in paperback) and the supplemental CD-ROM, along with sport-specific DVD training systems for golf, soccer, tennis, football, and baseball. Each of these DVDs contains a program with more than 60 exercises designed in a program to help you prepare to thrive in each of these sports. These are great products if you're a competitive or recreational athlete, and I have even recommended them with great success to professional athletes who cannot join us at our Athletes' Performance facilities.

I also recommend that you check out our powerful interactive platform, which can be accessed from www.coreperformance.com. We created this platform based on feedback from readers of the original *Core Performance* who were looking for more progressions to the workout. This interactive platform features Core Performance programs for every level of fitness and every major sport. My staff and I assembled these programs in a powerful database, all customized to your goals, interests, and life's demands based on simple questions that you answer.

There is a complete nutritional system that complements your customized training program, providing you with recommendations on meal timing and food choices as part of your customized "Perfect Day" routine. We have effective visual tools that let you track and monitor your progress. There are video clips of every exercise. And I try to provide you with daily tips and world-class content that reflect the constantly evolving research and development we do at Athletes' Performance every day.

In short, www.coreperformance.com is the next best thing to being here in person.

Ultimately, I want you to be members of the Core Performance online community for life, which is why we have made a full-year membership available for less than the monthly cost of a daily cup of coffee. This means that for the cost of a personal training session, you will have progressive programs that are based upon your accomplishments and that can change with you as your goals and demands change.

Even better, because you already have made a commitment to joining the Core community, I am providing you with a free 3-week trial to try out the site. From www.coreperformance.com, simply click on "Enter Your Access Code" and type in the following code: CPE20495. You'll have 3 weeks to sample the programs, check out all of the amazing tools on the site, and decide whether you want to become a member.

A further benefit of your interactive Web site membership—trial or actual—is that you can access our Video Library and view video clips of every exercise that is in the Core Performance Essentials program. For those people who are visually oriented (and I'm one of them), these videos will help you to see the proper form of every exercise from two different angles. And as you know, it is important to do these exercises correctly to maximize the gain.

However you proceed from here, I hope you do so as a centered self. Operate with core values, with long-term health as your first priority, and you'll find that your body will become the vehicle for your success with family, at work, and in everything you do. Remember to think of yourself as an athlete competing in the Game of Life.

Don't look at this new lifestyle as a short-term solution. This is not a home renovation, something with a beginning and an end.

By making this investment in yourself, you improve not only your health but also your mental and spiritual outlook. You become a better spouse, a better parent, a better sibling. That means the lives of your loved ones improve as well.

Earlier in the book, you heard from Janet Oja, who said that this program allowed her to "dream bigger." By mastering movements, eliminating pain, boosting energy, and fueling your body properly, you'll walk with a little more swagger and confidence. You'll glide through life, feeling like you can master anything.

For Janet, that meant rappelling into canyons and climbing out by whatever means necessary. What's the equivalent of that in your life? What challenge would you like to meet?

I've had great success supporting people in the pursuit of their dreams. Some of them are prominent sports figures, but many of them are people just like you who have reached spectacular goals. What I love most is being able to build my clients, to see them evolve and reach their goals.

We tend to keep score in this country with money. Whoever dies with the most toys wins, right? Wrong. The winner is the one who dies at a ripe old age, while still living an active lifestyle, having elevated others and built deep relationships along the way. I hope you'll keep score of your success within this program—whatever your definition of success might be—not just by how much weight you've lost or how you look in the mirror, but by how the quality of your life has improved. You've heard from people in this book who have lost weight, but the most important thing was that they found more energy for their children and significant others. And at Athletes' Performance, we've heard from others who have gained the confidence to pursue entrepreneurial endeavors, travel the world, or simply pursue a sport or physical activity that they never dared try before.

I'm excited about this book because I will get to hear from more people like you, and that inspires me. So many of you have become vocal advocates for this program, and I can't tell you how much I appreciate that.

I'm blown away when I hear someone like Mike Dixey tell me that he's used this program to overcome something like vertigo. Mike concluded his note with, "Mark, you have truly made a significant impact on my life. Anytime you have a bad day or need a lift, please pull out this letter and read it."

You bet I will, Mike.

I want to hear how this program has transformed your life—and not just from a physical standpoint. Tell me how it's enabled you to meet challenges and fulfill your dreams. I want to hear about what you've overcome and the roadblocks you've navigated. Tell the entire Core community how taking a proactive approach to life has made a difference.

Please share your stories with us at mark@coreperformance.com. We'll pick the most inspirational submissions, the ones that touch us the most, and bring the authors of those remarks to Athletes' Performance to train in person with our staff, alongside some of the best athletes in the world.

Let's help each other stay motivated through the Web site, where I will track your progress based upon your goals. You will empower me through your achievements and courage. You can share with me personally how you've transformed your life to meet your goals, motivating me even further.

We can't bring everyone out, unfortunately. I hope you join our online community and interact with the growing number of people dedicated to treating each day as an athletic event and properly preparing themselves for the competition that is the Game of Life.

Welcome to the Core.

Your coach,

Mark Verstegen

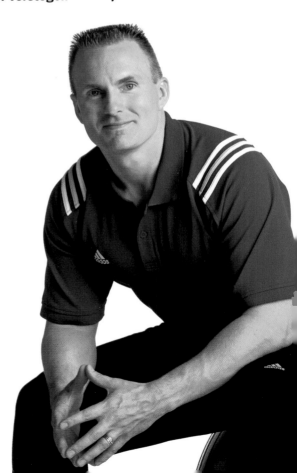

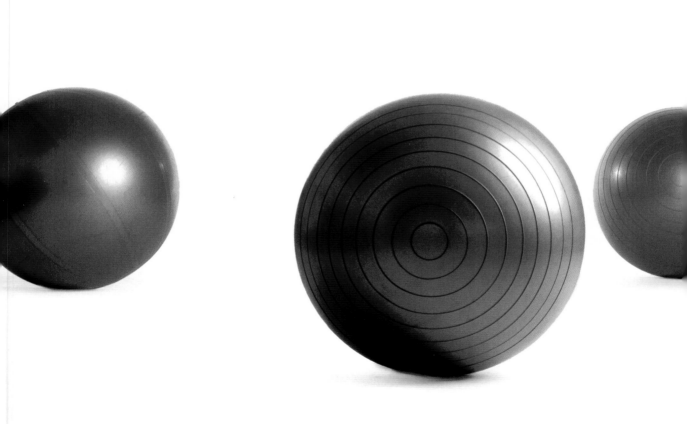

THE CORE WORKOUT AT A GLANCE

After my first book, *Core Performance,* we received a lot of suggestions from readers about how they would have preferred the exercises presented differently. Recognizing that people visualize and process information differently, we've laid out the exercises in three ways.

We've presented the Core Workout in a level-by-level format (pages 118 to 125) and in an exercise-by-exercise format (pages 126 to 178). With this appendix, I thought I'd combine the two and give you another at-a-glance view of the Core Workout. In all three versions, you'll see that while there are not that many exercises, the variations and progressions are virtually unlimited.

MOVEMENT PREP: HIP CROSS

90/90 STRETCH

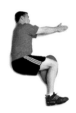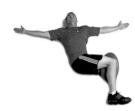

PROCEDURE: Lie on the ground on your left side in a fetal position, with your legs tucked up into your torso at a 90-degree angle and a pad or rolled-up towel between your knees. Keep both arms straight at a 90-degree angle to your torso. Now, keeping your knees together and on the ground and your hips still, rotate your chest and right arm back to the right, trying to put your back on the ground. Exhale and hold for 2 seconds, then return to the starting position. Finish your reps, then switch sides and repeat.

90/90 STRETCH (LEGS CROSSED)

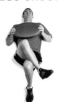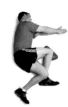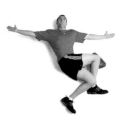

PROCEDURE: Lie faceup on the ground holding a pad or towel roll, your left knee bent to 90 degrees, and your right leg crossed over the left. Roll over onto your left side and pin a pad between your right knee and the ground. Maintaining pressure on the pad and keeping your hips still, rotate your chest and right arm back to the right, trying to put your back on the ground. Hold for 2 seconds, then return to the starting position. Repeat until you've completed your reps, then switch sides.

HIP CROSSOVER

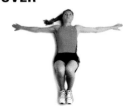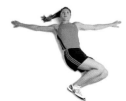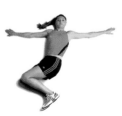

PROCEDURE: Lie faceup on the ground with your arms to your sides, your knees bent, and your feet flat. Twist your bent legs to the left until they reach the floor, then twist them to the right. Continue for the prescribed number of repetitions.

HIP CROSSOVER (FEET UP)

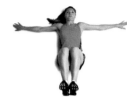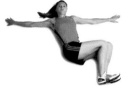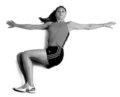

PROCEDURE: Try this move with your hips and knees bent 90 degrees and your feet off the ground. Once you master that, perform this move with your legs straight.

LUNGE STRETCH

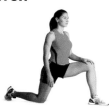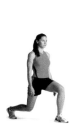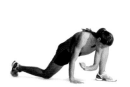

PROCEDURE: Take a half-step forward with your left foot, placing your right hand on the floor for balance. Take your left elbow and reach down your instep (on your forward leg). Place your left hand on the floor and push your hips upward as you straighten your front leg. Return to the starting position and repeat. **COACHING KEY:** Contract (squeeze) the glute muscle of your back leg. **YOU SHOULD FEEL:** A stretch through the groin, the hip flexor muscle of your back leg, the glute muscle of your front leg, and your hamstring.

LUNGE STRETCH (BACKWARD)

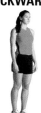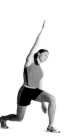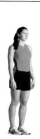

PROCEDURE: With your feet together, step back with your right leg into a lunge. While reaching your right hand to the sky, bend your torso to the left. Straighten your torso and step forward into the starting position. Alternate sides and repeat for the prescribed repetitions.

LUNGE STRETCH (MOVING)

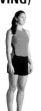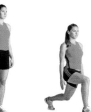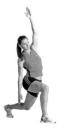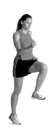

PROCEDURE: Instead of returning to the starting position as in Level 2, walk forward into the next position.

  209

INVERTED HAMSTRING (IN PLACE)

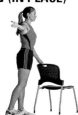
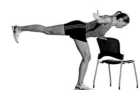

PROCEDURE: Stand on one leg with perfect posture, holding on to a wall, chair, or table for stability. Keep your shoulder blades back and down. Maintaining a straight line from ear to ankle, bend over at the waist, raising your opposite heel to the sky. When you feel a stretch, return to the standing position by contracting the muscles of your hamstring, glutes, and back. Complete your reps on that side, then switch legs. **COACHING KEY:** Keep your back flat and your hips and shoulders parallel to the ground. Maintain a straight line from your ear through your hip, knee, and ankle. Try to keep your balance without relying on your hand, and keep your opposite foot off the ground. **YOU SHOULD FEEL:** A stretch in your hamstrings.

INVERTED HAMSTRING (BACKWARD)

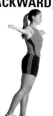
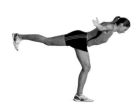

PROCEDURE: Step back into the next step and repeat using the opposite leg, alternating legs until you've completed all your reps.

MOVEMENT PREP: LATERAL LUNGE

LATERAL LUNGE

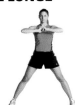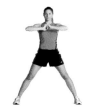

PROCEDURE: Standing with your feet wider than shoulder width apart, shift your hips to the left and down by bending your left knee and keeping your right leg straight. Your feet should be straight ahead and flat on the ground. Push through your left hip, returning to the starting position. Alternate sides and repeat for the prescribed number of repetitions. **COACHING KEY:** Keep your knee on your "working" side behind your toes. Keep your opposite leg straight, your back flat, and your chest up. **YOU SHOULD FEEL:** A lengthening and strengthening of your glutes, groin, hamstrings, and quads.

LATERAL LUNGE (STEP AND RETURN)

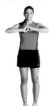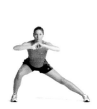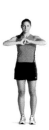

PROCEDURE: Step to the right with your right foot, keeping your toes forward and your feet flat. Squat through your right hip while keeping your left leg straight. Squat as low as possible, holding this position for 2 seconds. Push back to the starting position and repeat to the opposite side.

LATERAL LUNGE (MOVING)

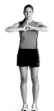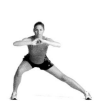

PROCEDURE: Instead of returning to the starting position, step into a squat position and then into the next lunge. Repeat for the prescribed number of repetitions and then switch sides. You will be stepping around the room during this exercise, so give yourself plenty of space.

L E V E L 2

HANDWALK (REVERSE)

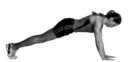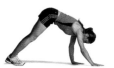

PROCEDURE: Bend at the waist and walk your feet out into a pushup position. Now, keeping your knees straight, walk your hands toward your feet. When you feel a stretch, walk your feet back out to a pushup position. Repeat until you've completed your reps. **COACHING KEY:** Keep your knees straight and your stomach tight. Walk your hands out farther beyond your head for increased difficulty. Use short "ankle steps" to walk back up to your hands. That is, take baby steps using only your ankles—don't use your knees, hips, or quads. **YOU SHOULD FEEL:** A stretch in your hamstrings, lower back, glutes, and calves.

L E V E L 3 & 4

HANDWALK

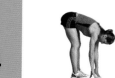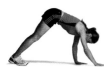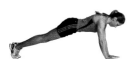

PROCEDURE: Instead of walking your feet back, walk your hands forward into a pushup position. Keeping your knees straight, walk your feet toward your hands until you feel a stretch in your hamstrings. Walk your hands forward to begin the next repetition. You will be moving around the room during this exercise, so give yourself plenty of space.

DROP LUNGE

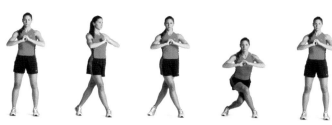

PROCEDURE: Reach your left foot 2 feet behind your right foot. Square your hips back to the starting position, and sit back and down into a squat. Stand and step laterally with your right foot, then repeat the stretch on the same side. Continue until you've completed your reps on that side, then reverse directions. **COACHING KEY:** Keep your chest up and sit your hips back. Maintain your weight on the heel of your front leg. You will be moving around the room during this exercise, so give yourself plenty of space. **YOU SHOULD FEEL:** A stretch in the outsides of both hips.

LEVEL 1

PILLAR BRIDGE FRONT (KNEELING)

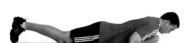

PROCEDURE: Lying on your stomach with your forearms on the ground under your chest, push off of your elbows, supporting your weight on your forearms and knees. Hold a static position for the prescribed length of time. Push your neck and sternum as far up and away from your forearms as possible. **COACHING KEY:** Keep your stomach tight. **YOU SHOULD FEEL IT:** In your shoulders and trunk.

LEVEL 2

PILLAR BRIDGE FRONT

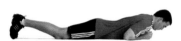

PROCEDURE: Same procedure as for Level 1, but instead of finishing with your knees on the floor, end in a prone pushup position, with just your forearms and toes resting on the floor. Push your chest as far away from the ground as possible. Hold your position for the prescribed amount of time. **COACHING KEY:** Keep your tummy tight and your head in line with your spine. There should be a straight line between your ear and your ankle, with no sagging or bending.

LEVEL 3

PILLAR BRIDGE FRONT (WIDE FEET)

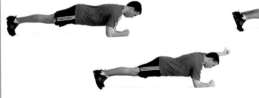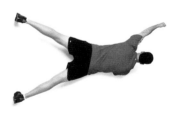

PROCEDURE: Lift one arm, hold for 2 seconds. Switch arms. Widen your feet, if necessary, to reduce difficulty.

LEVEL 4

PILLAR BRIDGE FRONT (NARROW FEET)

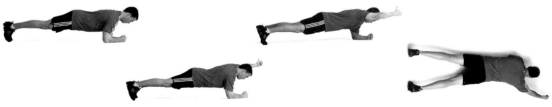

PROCEDURE: Same exercise as in Level 3. This time, narrow your feet to add to the degree of difficulty.

WWW.COREPERFORMANCE.COM

PILLAR BRIDGE LATERAL (KNEELING)

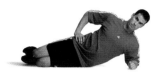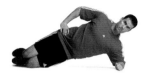

PROCEDURE: Lie on your side with your forearm on the ground and your elbow under your shoulder, with your knees bent to 90 degrees. Push your forearm away from your body, lifting your hips into the air and supporting your weight on your forearm and knees. Hold a static position for the prescribed amount of time. Complete the reps on one side, then switch. **COACHING KEY:** Keep your body in a straight line and keep your stomach tight. If this is too difficult, do individual repetitions—1 repetition per 2 seconds. **YOU SHOULD FEEL IT:** In your shoulders and trunk.

PILLAR BRIDGE LATERAL

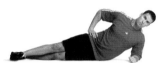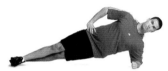

PROCEDURE: Lie on your side with your forearm on the ground under your shoulder, your feet split with the top leg forward. With your body in a straight line and your elbow under your shoulder, push your hip off the ground, creating a straight line from ankle to shoulder and keeping your head in line with your spine. Hold your position for the prescribed amount of time.

PILLAR BRIDGE LATERAL (STACKED FEET)

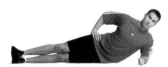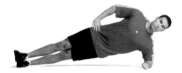

PROCEDURE: Instead of splitting your feet, stack them together.

PILLAR BRIDGE LATERAL (JUMPING JACK)

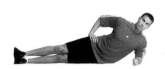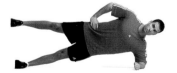

PROCEDURE: From the bridge position, lift your top leg into the air as if you were doing a lateral jumping jack.

L
E
V
E
L
1

GLUTE BRIDGE (MINI BAND)

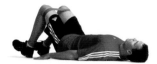
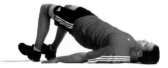

PROCEDURE: Place a mini band just above your knees. Lying faceup on the ground with your arms to your sides, your knees bent, and your heels on the ground, lift your hips off the ground until your knees, hips, and shoulders are in a straight line. Hold for the prescribed time. If this is too difficult, divide the time into 2- to 3-second intervals, then return to the starting position and repeat until you've completed all of your prescribed time. **COACHING KEY:** Fire (squeeze) your glutes. **YOU SHOULD FEEL IT:** In your glutes, and to a lesser degree in your hamstrings and lower back.

L
E
V
E
L
2

GLUTE BRIDGE (PADDED)

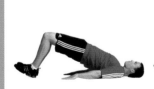
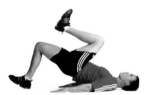

PROCEDURE: Squeeze a rolled-up towel, a doubled-over Thera-Band pad, or even a ball between your knees. Lift your hips into the air and then return to the starting position. Repeat for the prescribed number of reps.

L
E
V
E
L
3

GLUTE BRIDGE (MARCHING)

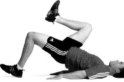
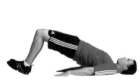

PROCEDURE: Try "marching" with one leg at a time.

L
E
V
E
L
4

GLUTE BRIDGE (KNEE BENT)

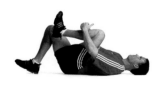
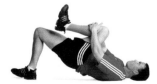

PROCEDURE: Try it with one leg held to your chest and your weight supported on the other leg. Switch legs.

MINI BAND STANDING

L
E
V
E
L
2

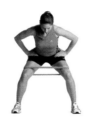 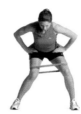

PROCEDURE: Stand with your feet just outside of your hips and a mini band above your knees. Take a partial squat. Keeping your left leg stationary, rotate your right knee in and out for the prescribed number of reps. Then switch legs and repeat. **COACHING KEY:** Keep both feet flat on the ground and your pelvis stable. Don't let the knee of your stationary leg drop in. **YOU SHOULD FEEL IT:** In your glutes.

MINI BAND WALKING

L
E
V
E
L
3

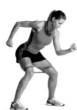 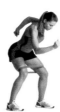 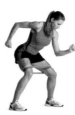

PROCEDURE: Move to the right, pushing with your left leg while stepping laterally with your right leg. Bring your left foot back to the starting position and continue until you've completed your reps on that side. Be sure to keep your knees pushed apart throughout the movement. Repeat while moving to the left.

MINI BAND WALKING (ADD RESISTANCE)

L
E
V
E
L
4

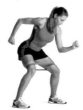 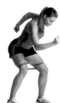 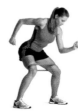

PROCEDURE: Increase the resistance by using a band with greater tension.

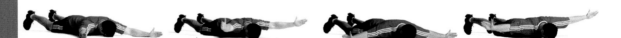

LEVEL 1

FLOOR Ys AND Ts

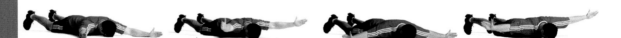

PROCEDURE: Lying facedown on the floor with your arms raised slightly above shoulder height, create a Y, with your torso and thumbs up. Glide your shoulder blades toward your spine and lift your arms off the ground. Return to the starting position and repeat to complete your reps. For the T, pull your shoulder blades in toward your spine and extend your arms to the sides to create a T with your torso. **COACHING KEY:** Keep your stomach tight and your thumbs up. Move from the scapulae (the shoulder blades), not from your arms, extending your shoulders and hands. **YOU SHOULD FEEL IT:** In your shoulders and upper back.

LEVEL 2

PHYSIOBALL Ys AND Ts (ARMS BENT)

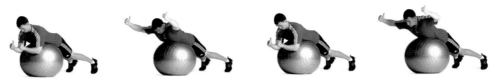

PROCEDURE: Perform the same exercise with bent elbows on a physioball, lying facedown over the top of the ball so that your back is flat and your chest is off the ball.

LEVEL 3

PHYSIOBALL Ys AND Ts (ARMS EXTENDED)

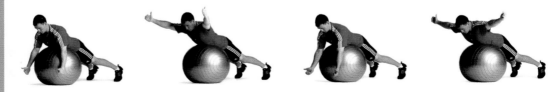

PROCEDURE: Perform the same exercise as for Level 2, but with your arms extended instead of bent.

LEVEL 4

PHYSIOBALL Ys AND Ts (WITH WEIGHT)

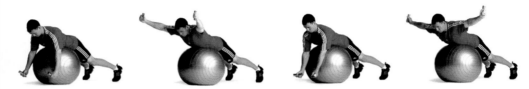

PROCEDURE: Add a light weight—1 to 3 pounds.

L E V E L 3

SUMO SQUAT TO HAMSTRING STRETCH

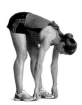 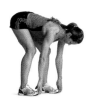

PROCEDURE: Standing with your feet shoulder width apart, bend at the waist and grab your toes. Drop your hips to the ground, lift your chest up, and then pull your hips forward until your torso is vertical. Maintaining a flat back, push your hips up and back until you feel a stretch in your hamstrings. Drop your hips back to the ground and repeat until you've completed all your reps. **COACHING KEY:** Keep your chest up, your back flat, and your heels on the floor. Keep your elbows inside of your knees. For an easier move, place a $\frac{1}{4}$- to 2-inch block under your heels. As your mobility and stability improve, perform the movement with a smaller and smaller heel lift. **YOU SHOULD FEEL:** A stretch in your hamstrings, groin, lower back, and quads.

PHYSIOBALL PLATE CRUNCH

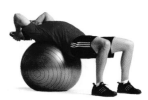 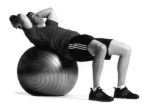

PROCEDURE: Lying on top of the ball, arch your torso over the ball. Try to touch your shoulder blades, back, and glutes over the ball so that your abdominals are completely stretched. Hold the weight plate behind your head. Roll your hips and chest up at the same time while pulling your belly button in. Crunch from the top of your torso and then lower your hips and chest to the starting position. **COACHING KEY:** Arch your torso completely. **YOU SHOULD FEEL:** A stretch in your abs and core.

LEVEL 2

PUSHUP (KNEELING)

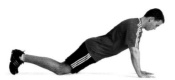
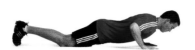

PROCEDURE: Assume a pushup position with your hands and knees on the ground. Lower your body to the ground, then reverse the movement without touching the ground. Keep your body in a straight line. **COACHING KEY:** Push your sternum as far away from your hands as possible at the end of the movement. **YOU SHOULD FEEL IT:** In your chest, arms, and torso.

LEVEL 2

PUSHUP

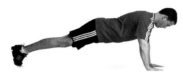
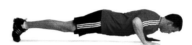

PROCEDURE: If you don't need to kneel, assume the normal pushup position.

LEVEL 3

PUSHUP (WITH PHYSIOBALL)

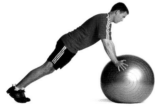
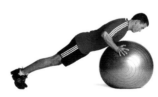

PROCEDURE: Assume a pushup position, but with your hands on a physioball and your feet on the floor. With your belly button drawn in, lower yourself to the point where your chest barely grazes the ball. Control the ball as you push back up, holding your belly button in and pushing your sternum as far away from the ball as possible. Your shoulder blades should be pushed away from each other in a "plus" position (as far forward as possible) at the top of the movement. Keep your fingers pointed down the sides of the ball.

GLUTE BRIDGE (WITH PHYSIOBALL)

LEVEL 2

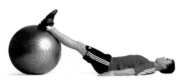 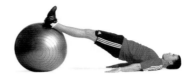

PROCEDURE: Lie faceup on the ground with your tummy tight and your feet on the ball (or on a bench or a couch). Your legs should be straight, your toes pulled up toward your shins, and your shoulder blades pulled back and down. Contract your glutes to raise your hips until you create a straight line between your ankle and shoulders, so that only your head, shoulders, and arms are touching the floor. Hold for 2 to 3 seconds and repeat until you've completed your reps. **COACHING KEY:** Initiate the movement by firing your glutes, and keep them contracted at the top of the movement. If it is too difficult to balance, spread your arms out to the side. Or, to make it more difficult, cross your arms on your chest. **YOU SHOULD FEEL IT:** In your glutes, hamstrings, and lower back.

GLUTE BRIDGE (WITH PHYSIOBALL LEG CURL)

LEVEL 3

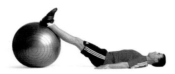 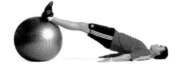 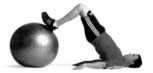

PROCEDURE: Contract your glutes to raise your hips, then pull your heels toward your body. Do not let your hips drop as the ball comes toward you. Extend your legs, then repeat the leg curl for the prescribed number of reps without letting your hips touch the ground.

222

FLOOR CRUNCH

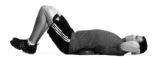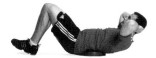

PROCEDURE: Lie faceup with your knees bent, with a small pad or towel under your lower back to help stretch your abs, and your hands behind your head supporting your neck. Lift your chest until your shoulder blades are off the ground, and at the same time rotate your pelvis toward your belly button. Slowly return to the starting position. Repeat until you've completed your reps. **COACHING KEY:** Do not pull on your head with your hands. Feel each segment of your spine flexing as you crunch and as you stretch over the pad. **YOU SHOULD FEEL IT:** In your abdominals.

PHYSIOBALL CRUNCH

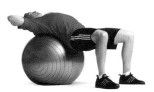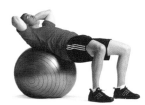

PROCEDURE: Lie faceup with your body arched over the ball and your hands interlocked, supporting your head. Drape your body over the ball—you should feel a mild stretch in your abs. Curl your trunk and pelvis together while keeping your belly button pulled in. Return to the starting position and repeat until you've completed all your reps.

SQUAT (BODY WEIGHT, WITH MINI BAND)

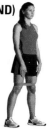
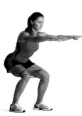

PROCEDURE: Stand with your arms at your sides, your feet shoulder width apart and pointing straight ahead, and a mini band around and above your knees. Maintain perfect posture and initiate movement with your hips. As you reach your arms far forward, squat your hips back and down until your thighs are parallel to the floor. Return to a standing position by pushing through your hips. Keep your knees out. Repeat until you've completed all your reps. **COACHING KEY:** Keep your knees behind your toes during the movement. Also, keep your knees pushing out against the band so that they do not collapse to the inside during the movement. If you extend your arms in front of you, you can sit back more comfortably. Keep your chest up and your back flat. **YOU SHOULD FEEL IT:** In your glutes, hamstrings, and quads.

SQUAT (SINGLE LEG)

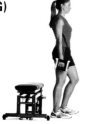
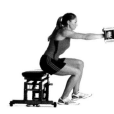
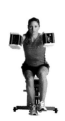

PROCEDURE: Stand on one foot in front of a bench or chair, holding 2½- to 5-pound weights in each hand. Initiate movement with your hips, squatting back and down on one leg as you reach forward until your glutes touch the bench. Return to a standing position using only the leg you are balancing on. Repeat for the prescribed number of repetitions, then switch legs. Do not let your knee collapse to the inside.

SPLIT SQUAT

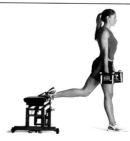
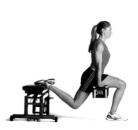

PROCEDURE: Hold dumbbells at arm's length at your sides. Place your back foot on a box or bench and step out into a lunge. Lower your hips toward the floor by squatting back and down. Without letting your back knee touch the ground, return to the starting position by driving your weight back up with your front leg. Do all the reps with that leg forward, then switch legs and repeat. **COACHING KEY:** Don't let your front knee slide forward over your toes; if it does, start over again with your front foot farther forward. **YOU SHOULD FEEL IT:** In your hips and the fronts of your legs.

SPLIT DUMBBELL CURL

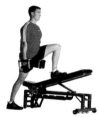 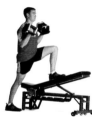

PROCEDURE: In a standing position, hold dumbbells at your side and place one leg on a stable object at about midthigh height. Shift your weight forward onto your front leg, taking your back leg into a stretch. Now, keeping your elbows still, lift the dumbbells to your shoulders as you rotate your palms to the ceiling. Return to the starting position and repeat until you've completed all your reps. Switch legs midway through the set. **COACHING KEY:** Keep your stomach and the glute muscles of your rear leg tight throughout the movement. Do not allow your back to move. Do not rock forward or backward, and don't move your elbows. **YOU SHOULD FEEL IT:** In your biceps, glutes, and hip flexors.

SPLIT DUMBBELL CURL TO PRESS

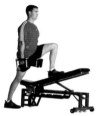 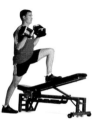 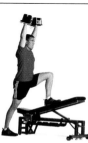

PROCEDURE: After performing a biceps curl, press the weight over your head, finishing with your palms facing forward. Switch legs midway through the set.

ALTERNATING SPLIT DUMBBELL CURL TO PRESS

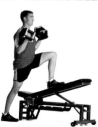 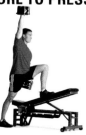 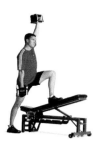

PROCEDURE: Stand holding dumbbells at your sides with your front foot resting on a bench or sturdy step at about midthigh height. Push your body weight slightly forward, with your back glute tight. Perform a biceps curl so that the dumbbells are at your chest. Press your right hand over your head as you lower the left. As you lower your right hand, repeat the motion with your left arm so that the dumbbells pass at your torso. Repeat for the prescribed number of repetitions, switching the foot on the bench halfway through the set. Contract the glute of your back leg to stabilize yourself. Switch legs midway through the set. **COACHING KEY:** Maintain perfect posture, with your belly button pulled in and your shoulder blades pulled back and down. Do not let your back arch when the weight is pressed overhead. **YOU SHOULD FEEL IT:** In your biceps and shoulders, and throughout your pillar.

STANDING LIFT

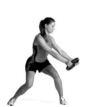
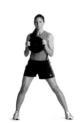
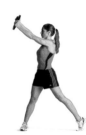

PROCEDURE: Squat, rotating from left to right while holding a weight plate. Square up and press the plate over your head. **COACHING KEY:** Keep your chest up and your back flat. This exercise combines the familiar movements of squatting, rotating, the upright row, and the incline press. Lower in the same pattern as you lifted. **YOU SHOULD FEEL IT:** In your hips, torso rotators, upper back, chest, and shoulders.

STANDING LIFT (ONE LEG)

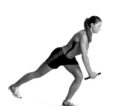
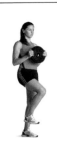
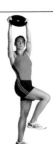

PROCEDURE: Stand holding a weight plate or dumbbell in a low position, or holding a rope handle attached to a low pulley cable. Your foot should be perpendicular to the cable if you are using one, your hips should be flexed, and your abdominals should be drawn in. Balance on your inside foot, turn your shoulders and hip toward the leg that's supporting your weight, and keep your chest up and your stomach tight. Squat down so that the weight is outside this leg, then fire from your glutes and torso. Pull the weight or handles toward your chest while extending your supporting leg. Turn your trunk away from your supporting leg as your hands push up and away. Return to the starting position and repeat to complete your reps, then switch legs. **COACHING KEY:** Keep your chest up and your back flat. Your torso will rotate from start to finish. This exercise combines the familiar movements of balance squatting, rotating, the upright row, and the incline press. Lower in the same pattern as you lifted. **YOU SHOULD FEEL IT:** In your hips, torso rotators, upper back, chest, and shoulders.

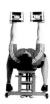

ALTERNATING DUMBBELL BENCH PRESS

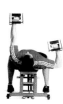 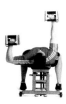 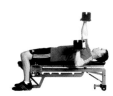

PROCEDURE: Lie faceup on a bench, holding dumbbells at the outside edges of your shoulders, your palms facing your thighs. Lift the dumbbells straight up over your chest. Keeping one arm straight, lower the other dumbbell, touch the outside of your shoulder, then push it back up. Switch arms and continue to alternate arms for the prescribed number of repetitions. **COACHING KEY:** Keep your nonworking arm straight. Keep your feet on the floor and your hips and shoulders on the bench at all times. Pull your stomach in to stabilize your core. **YOU SHOULD FEEL IT:** In your chest, shoulders, and triceps.

ROMANIAN DEADLIFT (TWO ARMS, ONE LEG)

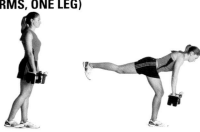

PROCEDURE: Stand on one foot while holding a dumbbell in each hand, using an overhand grip. "Hinge" over at the waist, lowering the dumbbells as your nonsupporting leg lifts behind you. Return to the standing position by contracting your hamstrings and glutes. Repeat for the prescribed number of repetitions, then switch legs. **COACHING KEY:** Do not let your back arch. Your torso and leg should move as one unit. Fire the glute of your extended leg to keep it straight. Keep your shoulder blades back and down throughout the movement, and keep the dumbbells close to your shin. **YOU SHOULD FEEL IT:** In your glutes, hamstrings, and back.

ONE-ARM, ONE-LEG DUMBBELL ROW

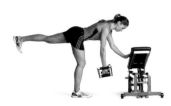 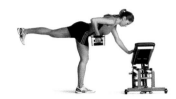

PROCEDURE: Stand on your right leg, hinged over at the waist, holding a dumbbell with your right hand and holding on to a stable, waist-high surface with your left hand. Lift your left leg to form a *T* with your body. Slide your right shoulder blade toward your spine and then lift the weight to your body by driving your elbow to the ceiling. Return to the starting position and repeat for the prescribed number of repetitions. Then switch sides. **COACHING KEY:** Move with your shoulder, not your arm, to initiate the row. Keep your back level—your shoulders should stay parallel to the floor—and fire the glute of your extended leg to keep it parallel to the floor. Extend the leg opposite the hand doing the lifting. **YOU SHOULD FEEL IT:** In your back, lats, and shoulders.

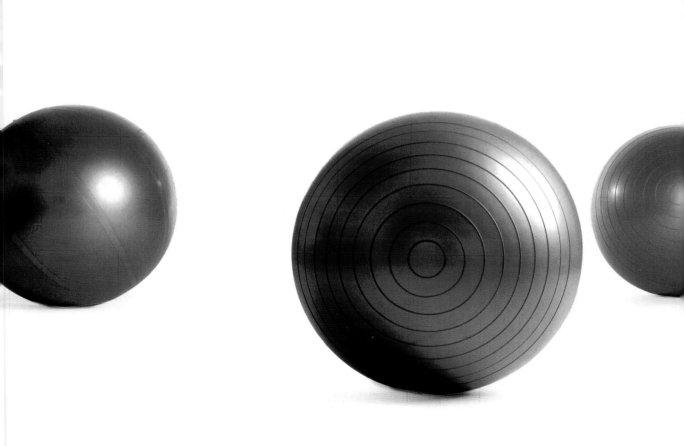

ACKNOWLEDGMENTS

Writing a book, like the Game of Life, is a team effort. This book would not have been completed were it not for a talented team of people playing their positions exceptionally well.

That team could fill the largest locker room, and space prohibits me from thanking everyone by name. I must, however, single out the staff, athletes, and extended family of Athletes' Performance for their input and inspiration. Special thanks go to Amanda Carlson, Craig Friedman, and Dan Burns for helping to shape the message of this program. I am also grateful for the insights from our friends at Tignum (www.tignum.com), namely Hans-Jürgen Rippel and Scott Peltin. Debbie Martell, the wonderful performance chef at Athletes' Performance, provided a huge assist with the recipes in this book. As always, I owe a huge debt of gratitude to my co-conspirators David Black and Pete Williams, along with Rodale's team of Jeremy Katz, Pete Fornatale, Susan Eugster, Karen Neely, Susannah Hogendorn, and Jennifer Giandomenico for helping me fulfill the goal of sharing the Core message with others. Last of all to my beautiful wife, Amy; our family; and our Athletes' Performance team.

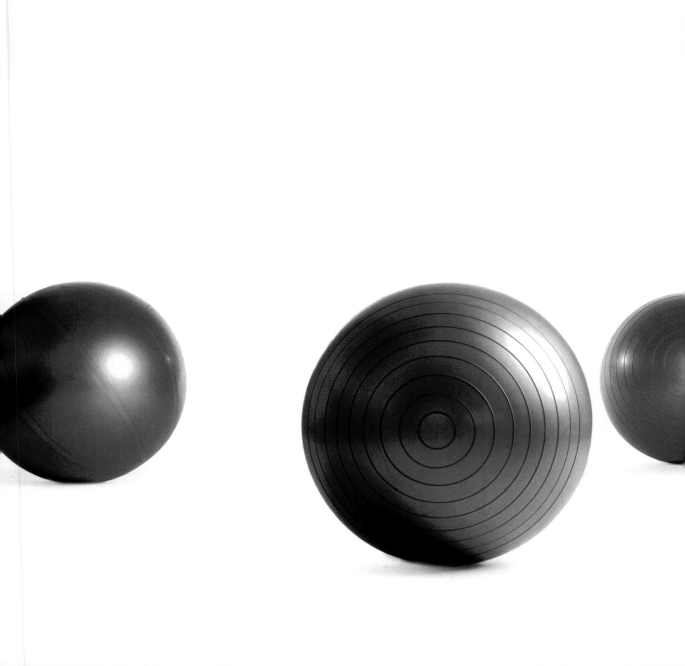

INDEX

Boldface page references indicate photographs and illustrations.
Underscored references indicate boxed text.

ABOUT THE AUTHORS

Mark Verstegen is recognized as one of the world's most innovative sports performance experts. As the owner of Athletes' Performance—cutting-edge training centers in Tempe, Arizona, and Carson, California—he directs teams of performance specialists and nutritionists to train some of the most recognized names in sports.

By teaching an integrated lifestyle and training program that blends strength, speed, flexibility, joint and "core" stability, and mental toughness, Verstegen helps athletes become not only faster and stronger but also more powerful, flexible, and resistant to injury and long-term back, hip, and other joint problems.

Because of his innovative techniques and up-to-date knowledge of sports performance, Verstegen is a sought-after consultant. He serves as director of performance for the NFL Players Association, is an advisor to Adidas, EAS, Amino Vital, and other leading performance-oriented companies, and serves as a consultant to numerous athletic governing bodies.

A dynamic speaker, Verstegen travels the world to address groups such as the American College of Sports Medicine, the National Strength and Conditioning Association, and many corporate audiences.

Verstegen and his training methods have been profiled by dozens of national media outlets. He's a contributing columnist to *Men's Health*® magazine and the executive producer of fitness programs for Sportskool, the nation's first video-on-demand cable network dedicated to expert sports and fitness instruction. His first book, *Core Performance: The Revolutionary Workout Program to Transform Your Body and Your Life,* was published by Rodale in 2004 and soared to as high as No. 24 on the Amazon.com best-seller list.

Verstegen began his coaching career at his alma mater, Washington State University, following a career-ending football injury. He served as assistant director of player development at Georgia Tech and in 1994 created the International Performance Institute on the campus of the IMG Sports Academy in Bradenton, Florida. In 1999, he moved to Phoenix to build Athletes' Performance, which quickly became the industry leader for training world-class athletes.

Verstegen and his wife, Amy, live in Scottsdale, Arizona.

Pete Williams is a veteran journalist who has written about sports, business, and fitness for numerous publications, including *USA Today,* the *Washington Post,* and Street & Smith's *SportsBusiness Journal.* He is the author of two books on the sports memorabilia business—*Card Sharks* and *Sports Memorabilia for Dummies*—and is coauthor of two previous Rodale books: *Core Performance* (with Mark Verstegen) and *Fun Is Good* (with Mike Veeck). A graduate of the University of Virginia, he lives in Florida with his wife, Suzy, and sons, Luke and Lance.

For more information on Mark Verstegen's Core training programs, including interactive workouts and nutritional plans, please visit www.coreperformance.com. The site also offers sport-specific, DVD programs for tennis, golf, soccer, baseball, football, and other sports, along with Core training equipment and information on how to attend seminars and personalized training weeks at Athletes' Performance in Tempe, Arizona, and Carson, California.

For more information on Pete Williams, please visit www.petewilliams.net.